Transitions of Care in Pharmacy Casebook

Transitions of Care in Pharmacy Casebook

Editors

Laressa Bethishou, PharmD, APh, BCPS

Assistant Professor of Pharmacy Practice
Chapman University School of Pharmacy
Irvine, California

Jessica Wooster, PharmD, BCACP

Clinical Assistant Professor
Ben and Maytee Fisch College of Pharmacy
University of Texas at Tyler
Tyler, Texas

Phung C. On, PharmD, BCPS

Assistant Professor of Pharmacy Practice
School of Pharmacy
Massachusetts College of Pharmacy and Health Sciences
Boston, Massachusetts

New York   Chicago   San Francisco   Athens   London   Madrid   Mexico City
Milan   New Delhi   Singapore   Sydney   Toronto

Transitions of Care in Pharmacy Casebook

1 2 3 4 5 6 7 8 9 LOV 26 25 24 23 22 21

ISBN 978-1-260-47461-9
MHID 1-260-47461-5

This book was set in Minion Pro by MPS Limited.
The editors were Michael Weitz and Peter J. Boyle.
The production supervisor was Catherine H. Saggese.
Project management was provided by Jyoti Shaw, MPS Limited.

This book is printed on acid-free paper.

Library of Congress Cataloging-in-Publication Data
Names: Bethishou, Laressa, editor. | Wooster, Jessica, editor. | On, Phung C., editor.
Title: Transitions of care in pharmacy casebook / editors, Laressa Bethishou, Jessica Wooster, Phung C. On.
Description: New York : McGraw Hill, [2021] | Includes bibliographical references and index. | Summary: "This text provide complex clinical cases which will incorporate specific elements of patient care which mimic real-world practice. Unlike many pharmacotherapy cases, these cases can be used by pharmacy instructors to prompt discussion, illicit critical thinking and to illustrate the specific needs of various patient populations and health conditions during transitions of care across health care settings"— Provided by publisher.
Identifiers: LCCN 2021005462 (print) | LCCN 2021005463 (ebook) | ISBN 9781260474619 (paperback) | ISBN 9781260474626 (ebook)
Subjects: MESH: Pharmaceutical Services | Continuity of Patient Care | Drug Therapy | Case Reports | Problems and Exercises
Classification: LCC RA975.5.P5 (print) | LCC RA975.5.P5 (ebook) | NLM QV 18.2 | DDC 362.17/82—dc23
LC record available at https://lccn.loc.gov/2021005462
LC ebook record available at https://lccn.loc.gov/2021005463

CONTENTS

CONTRIBUTORS

Laressa Bethishou, PharmD, APh, BCPS
Assistant Professor of Pharmacy Practice, Chapman
University School of Pharmacy, Irvine, California
Chapters 1, 3, 5, 11, 16, 17, 21

Don Branam, PharmD, BCPS, FASHP
Associate Professor of Pharmacy Practice, South College
School of Pharmacy, Knoxville, Tennessee
Chapter 21

Rachel A. Bratteli, PharmD, BCACP
Clinical Assistant Professor, Ben and Maytee Fisch College
of Pharmacy, University of Texas at Tyler, Tyler, Texas
Chapter 9

Danielle M. Candelario, PharmD, BCPS
Associate Professor, College of Pharmacy, Rosalind Franklin
University of Medicine and Science, North Chicago,
Illinois
Chapter 7

Elizabeth A. Cook, PharmD, AE-C, BCACP, CDE
Clinical Pharmacist Specialist, Robert J. Dole Veteran
Affairs Medical Center, Wichita, Kansas
Chapter 15

Rebecca L. Dunn, Pharm.D., BCPS
Clinical Associate Professor, Department of Clinical
Sciences, Ben and Maytee Fisch College of Pharmacy,
The University of Texas at Tyler, Tyler, Texas
Chapter 13

Erika Felix-Getzik, PharmD
Professor of Pharmacy Practice, School of Pharmacy –
Boston, MCPHS University, Boston, Massachusetts
Chapter 14

Jeffrey Gonzales, PharmD, PDE-C
Clinical Pharmacy Specialist, Transitions of Care,
St. Mary Medical Center, Langhorne, Pennsylvania
Chapter 17

Elizabeth Haftel, PharmD, CDE
Assistant Professor of Pharmacy Practice, School of
Pharmacy – Boston, MCPHS University, Boston,
Massachusetts
Chapter 10

Kristen Herzik, PharmD, BCPS
Assistant Professor of Clinical Sciences, Touro University
California College of Pharmacy, San Diego, California
Chapter 3

Jelena Lewis, PharmD, APh, BCACP
Assistant Professor of Pharmacy Practice, Chapman
University School of Pharmacy, Irvine, California
Chapter 11

Rupal Mansukhani, PharmD, CTTS, FAPhA
Clinical Associate Professor, Ernest Mario School of
Pharmacy, Rutgers University, Piscataway, New Jersey
Chapter 18

Luma Munjy, PharmD
Assistant Professor of Pharmacy Practice, Chapman
University School of Pharmacy, Irvine, California
Chapter 17

Phung C. On, PharmD, BCPS
Assistant Professor of Pharmacy Practice, School of
Pharmacy – Boston, MCPHS University, Boston,
Massachusetts
Chapters 1, 2, 10, 12, 14, 20

Brittany L. Parmentier, PharmD, MPH, BCPS, BCPP
Clinical Assistant Professor, Ben and Maytee Fisch College of
Pharmacy, The University of Texas at Tyler, Tyler, Texas
Chapter 22

Khyati Patel, PharmD, BCACP
Ambulatory Care Pharmacist, Aurora Medical Center
Kenosha; Assistant Professor, College of Pharmacy,
Rosalind Franklin University of Medicine and Science,
North Chicago, Illinois
Chapter 7

Justin P. Reinert, PharmD, BCCCP
Clinical Assistant Professor, Ben and Maytee Fisch College of
Pharmacy, The University of Texas at Tyler, Tyler, Texas
Chapter 21

Nikhil A. Sangave, PharmD
Assistant Professor of Pharmacy Practice, School of
Pharmacy – Boston, MCPHS University, Boston,
Massachusetts
Chaptesr 12, 20

Winter J. Smith, PharmD, BCPS
Clinical Professor, Department of Clinical Sciences, Ben and
Maytee Fisch College of Pharmacy, The University
of Texas at Tyler, Tyler, Texas
Chapter 13

Roxane L. Took, PharmD, BCACP
Assistant Professor, Pharmacy Practice, St. Louis College
of Pharmacy, St. Louis, Missouri
Chapter 6

Laura Tsu, PharmD, BCPS, BCGP

Associate Professor of Pharmacy Practice Chapman
University School of Pharmacy Irvine, California
Chapter 16

Amulya Uppala, PharmD, BCPS

Clinical Pharmacist- Transitions of Care, Overlook
Medical Center, Summit, New Jersey
Chapter 8

Takova D. Wallace-Gay, PharmD, BCACP

Clinical Assistant Professor, Ben and Maytee Fisch College of
Pharmacy, The University of Texas at Tyler, Tyler, Texas
Chapter 9

Kimberly Won, PharmD, APh, BCCCP

Assistant Professor of Pharmacy Practice, Chapman
University School of Pharmacy, Irvine, California
Chapter 11

Jessica Wooster, PharmD, BCACP

Clinical Assistant Professor, The University of Texas at Tyler,
Ben and Maytee Fisch College of Pharmacy, Tyler, Texas
Chapters 1, 4, 5, 13, 15, 19, 22

Tianrui Yang, PharmD, BCPS

Clinical Assistant Professor, University of Texas at Tyler,
Tyler, Texas
Chapter 19

The Centers for Medicare & Medicaid Services (CMS) define a transition of care as the movement of a patient from one setting of care to another. Healthcare transitions can include a change in service or level of care, a change in setting, or a change in provider.[1] Ineffective transitions of care have consequences, including medication error and adverse events, excessive emergency department (ED) visits and avoidable readmissions, high costs to the healthcare system, and patient dissatisfaction.[2] Among Medicare patients, almost 20% who are discharged from a hospital are readmitted within 30 days. Unplanned readmissions, at a cost of $17.4 billion, accounted for 17% of total hospital payments from Medicare in 2004.[1]

There is both a need and an opportunity to promote safe and effective transitions of care as patients navigate through the healthcare system. This requires an interdisciplinary approach to care, improved collaboration between healthcare providers, and implementing interventions that aim to reduce medication errors and adverse events. Goals of transitions-of-care interventions include reducing hospital length of stay and avoidable readmissions, decreasing cost to the patient and healthcare system, and improving patient satisfaction.[2,3]

The pharmacist plays a valuable role in supporting transitions of care through his or her involvement in medication reconciliation, patient education, comprehensive discharge planning, and follow-up care coordination.[2,3] A multitude of published studies support pharmacist involvement in transitional care management of patients, and these efforts result in a reduction of overall and medication-related hospitalizations and ED visits. Other benefits elucidated in the studies include fewer preventable adverse drug events within 30 days of discharge, fewer medication discrepancies at discharge, and improved patient adherence and understanding of medication therapy.[4,5]

HOW TO USE THIS BOOK: STUDENTS

High-risk patient populations, including the elderly and those with multiple comorbidities, often benefit most from transitions-of-care interventions. This casebook will prompt students to apply principles of transitions of care in the provision of patient care across different disease states and healthcare settings. With each patient case, students should apply evidence-based medicine and guidelines to provide patient care, while considering patient needs based on the healthcare setting where care is being provided and as they transition to other settings of care (e.g., being discharged from the hospital to home versus to a long-term care facility). Students should apply the Pharmacists' Patient Care Process (PPCP) and collect, assess, plan, implement, and follow up while incorporating pharmacist interventions during transitions of care. As students answer questions, they should consider their rationale for why the selected answer was most appropriate given the unique needs of their patient.

HOW TO USE THIS BOOK: FACULTY

Faculty can assign patient cases and questions to students through the written text or online version available on Access Pharmacy (accesspharmacy.mhmedical.com). Answer rationales can be provided to faculty upon request. We encourage faculty to prompt students to provide their rationale for selected answers and discuss why their choices are most appropriate given their patients' unique needs at each setting during their transition of care.

REFERENCES

1. Centers for Medicare & Medicaid Services. Community-based care transitions program. Available at https://innovation.cms.gov/initiatives/CCTP. Accessed July 29, 2020.
2. American Pharmacists Association. Transitions of Care Toolkit. December 2019.
3. American Pharmacists Association. Applying the Pharmacists' Patient Care Process to Care Transitions Services. February 2019.
4. American College of Clinical Pharmacy, Hume AL, Kirwin J, Bieber HL, Couchenour RL, Hall DL, Kennedy AK, et al. Improving care transitions: current practice and future opportunities for pharmacists. *Pharmacotherapy*. 2012;32(11):e326-e337.
5. American College of Clinical Pharmacy, et al. Process indicators of quality clinical pharmacy services during transitions of care. *Pharmacotherapy*. 2012;32(11):e338-e347.

Section 1

Introduction to Transitions of Care Practice Models

1 Applying the Pharmacist Patient Care Process to Care Transitions

Laressa Bethishou   Phung C. On

Jessica Wooster

BACKGROUND

The Pharmacists' Patient Care Process (PPCP) provides a consistent process for delivery of care across the pharmacy profession. This process is applicable to any pharmacist practice setting and incorporates a patient-centered and interprofessional collaborative approach to optimizing patient care. Pharmacists use evidence-based principles to collect, assess, plan, implement, and provide follow-up care. These patient care activities are then communicated to the appropriate personnel (e.g., patient, primary care provider) and documented in the patient's health record to ensure continuity of care.[1,2]

As patients navigate through the healthcare system, there is a need and an opportunity to improve healthcare transitions. The Centers for Medicare & Medicaid Services (CMS) defines care transitions as the movement of a patient from one provider, or setting of care, to another.[3] With each care transition, patients may experience changes to their health status and medications, creating the potential for adverse events. Pharmacists are well poised to improve healthcare outcomes and reduce costs associated with ineffective patient hand-offs during transitions of care. Application of the PPCP to the provision of care transition services can maximize the pharmacist's role as a valuable member of the healthcare team.

When providing transitional care services, consider the following unique patient-specific considerations in applying the PPCP.

Collect

The pharmacist ensures the collection of necessary information to provide safe and effective transition of care (TOC). To guide clinical decision-making and medication therapy optimization, the pharmacist requires relevant health data and lifestyle information which supports TOC activities such as medication reconciliation, patient counseling, medication access or dispensing services, and post-discharge follow-up and monitoring. In addition to medical history, this may include collecting information on adherence barriers, educational deficits, level of independence, and caregiver support. Sources of information may include patient and caregiver interviews, electronic health records, and pharmacy or health facility records. Multiple sources should be utilized, as each source may have limitations.

Assess

The pharmacist will assess medications for appropriate indication, effectiveness, safety, and adherence. Clinical decision-making should consider past and current medical history, patient health status, changes to symptoms and labs, and any social, economic, or educational barriers to adherence. Medication therapy problems which may require intervention include unnecessary medication therapy, errors of omission, ineffective or duplicative therapy, incorrect dosages, need for additional monitoring, adverse events and drug interactions, and cost or adherence barriers.

Equally important, pharmacists should also assess the patient's medical condition(s) beyond what is needed for medication management. In addition to evaluating acute and chronic conditions for disease progression and improvement, pharmacists should assess for preventative care in order to help patients stay healthy.

Plan

The pharmacist will develop a plan, in collaboration with the patient and their healthcare team, for actions to be taken to identify and resolve medication problems, medication access issues, and low health literacy. An effective patient-centered care plan should address medication-related problems and optimize medication therapy, set goals of therapy for achieving clinical outcomes in the context of the patient's overall healthcare goals and access to care, engage the patient through education, empowerment, and self-management, and support care continuity, including follow-up and transitions of care as appropriate.

Implement

The pharmacist will implement the patient-centered care plan to optimize medication therapy during transitions of care. This includes addressing barriers to safe and effective transitions of care, management of acute and chronic disease states, providing education and self-management training, and supporting continuity of care.

Follow-Up: Monitor and Evaluate

The pharmacist will monitor and evaluate the effectiveness of the care plan. This includes evaluating medication appropriateness, effectiveness, and safety as well as patient adherence, outcomes of care, and progress toward achievement of goals of therapy. Modification of the plan may be required in collaboration with other healthcare professionals and the patient or caregiver.

At each care transition, the PPCP can be applied to optimize the provision of care. Pharmacists should collect relevant information to support formulating and implementing an assessment, plan, and follow-up which provide continuity of care and address patient specific needs.

PATIENT PRESENTATION

Chief Complaint

Epigastric pain and vomiting

History of Present Illness

MB is a 65-year-old Caucasian female who presented to the emergency department (ED) with epigastric pain and vomiting coffee ground—like substance. She reports tarry-looking stools and complains of having epigastric pain, most commonly after meals, over the last month. She takes Alka Seltzer to help with the stomach pain. MB has also been taking ibuprofen for back pain regularly, since she had a fall 2 months ago.

Past Medical History

Suspected peptic ulcer
Back pain
Depression

Surgical History

None

Family History

None

Social History

Patient is widowed and lives alone. She was brought in by her daughter.
She is a retired accountant.
She does not smoke or drink.

Immunization

Annual influenza vaccine

Insurance

Blue Cross Medicare Advantage

Allergies

No known allergies

Home Medications

- Alka Seltzer 1 tablet PO daily
- Fluoxetine 20 mg 1 tablet PO daily
- Ibuprofen 600 mg 1 tablet twice a day

Physical Examination

▸ **General**

Denies fever, chills, night sweats, weight loss.

▸ **HEENT**

Denies vision changes, vertigo, congestion, sore throat.

▸ **Cardiovascular**

Denies chest pain, palpitations, orthopnea, edema.

▸ **Respiratory**

Denies wheezing, cough or hemoptysis.

▸ **Gastrointestinal**

+ Epigastric pain, denies constipation, diarrhea, or change in frequency.

▸ **Urinary**

Denies dysuria, hematuria, urgency, or incontinence.

▸ **Musculoskeletal**

Lower back pain secondary to fall.

▸ **Neurologic**

Increased confusion; denies head injury/falls, numbness, tingling, or dizziness.

▸ **Psychological**

+ Depression, + insomnia.

Laboratory Findings

Na = 141 mEq/L	RBC = 4.7 × 10³/mm³	Ca = 8.1 mg/dL
K = 4.8 mEq/L	WBC = 9.2 10³/mm³	Mg = 2.4 mg/dL
Cl = 101 mEq/L	HCT = 34%	Phos = 4.8 mg/dL
CO_2 = 24 mEq/L	Plt = 130 × 10³/mm³	Hbg = 12.2 g/dL
SCr = 0.8 mg/dL		AST = 24 IU/L
BUN = 42 mg/dL		ALT = 32 IU/L
Glucose = 102 mg/dL		

QUESTIONS

1. When collecting a best possible medication history (BPMH) for the patient, which of the following is the preferred source of information?
   A. The patient
   B. The patient's daughter
   C. The patient's pharmacy records
   D. The patient's primary care physician

2. What is the most likely cause of the patient's suspected peptic ulcer?
   A. *Helicobacter pylori* infection
   B. Stress
   C. Weight gain
   D. Nonsteroidal anti-inflammatory drugs (NSAIDs) use

3. In addition to the information we have already collected for the patient, which of the following information is most important to the assessment and plan?
   A. The patient has an inpatient order for "nothing by mouth"
   B. The patient takes Tylenol PM 1 tablet by mouth at bedtime because she has trouble sleeping
   C. The patient takes her fluoxetine at night with dinner
   D. All of the above

4. The ED physician asks you for a recommendation for the management of MB's epigastric pain. Which of the following therapy options is the most appropriate?
   A. Famotidine 20 mg PO q12h
   B. Famotidine 20 mg IV q12h
   C. Pantoprazole 40 mg PO daily
   D. Pantoprazole 40 mg IV bid

5. The patient is now ready for discharge and will require a prescription for a proton pump inhibitor (PPI). In order to write the appropriate number of refills on the prescription, you must determine how long the patient needs to be on the PPI. Which of the following is the appropriate minimum duration of therapy for the treatment of noncardiac chest pain?
   A. 2 weeks
   B. 4 weeks
   C. 8 weeks
   D. Indefinitely

6. The patient has received her annual influenza vaccine but states she has not had any other vaccines since she was a child. The ED physician wants to make sure MB's vaccinations are up to date prior to discharge. What vaccines are indicated for MB based on her age and medical conditions?
   A. Zostavax and Pneumovax
   B. Zostavax and Prevnar 13
   C. Shingrix and Pneumovax
   D. Shingrix and Prevnar 13

7. Which of the following patient education points is most appropriate to discuss with the patient prior to discharge?
   A. Discontinue her fluoxetine as this medication is contributing to her difficulty sleeping
   B. Educate the patient to replace Tylenol PM with a prescription sleep aid
   C. Educate the patient to stop taking Alka Seltzer
   D. All of the above

8. At the patient's post-discharge follow-up appointment, which of the following should be assessed?
   A. Efficacy of her PPI
   B. Indication for calcium supplementation
   C. Management of her back pain
   D. All of the above

REFERENCES

1. Joint Commission of Pharmacy Practitioners. Pharmacists' Patient Care Process. Available at https://jcpp.net/wp-content/uploads/2016/03/PatientCareProcess-with-supporting-organizations.pdf. May 29, 2014.
2. American Pharmacists Association. Applying the Pharmacists' Patient Care Process to Care Transitions Services. February 2019.
3. Community-based care transitions program for Medicare and Medicaid Services. Available at https://innovation.cms.gov/initiatives/CCTP/. Accessed May 30, 2020.
4. By the 2019 American Geriatrics Society Beers Criteria® Update Expert Panel. American Geriatrics Society 2019 Updated AGS Beers Criteria® for Potentially Inappropriate Medication Use in Older Adults. *J Am Geriatr Soc.* 2019;67(4):674-694.
5. Schey R, Villarreal A, Fass R. Noncardiac chest pain: current treatment. *Gastroenterol Hepatol (N Y).* 2007;3(4):255-262.
6. Centers for Disease Control and Prevention. Vaccines and Immunizations. Available at https://www.cdc.gov/vaccines/index.html. May 26, 2016.
7. Jaynes M, Kumar AB. The risks of long-term use of proton pump inhibitors: a critical review. *Ther Adv Drug Saf.* 2018;10:2042098618809927. November 19, 2018.

2 Medication Reconciliation Best Practices

Phung C. On

BACKGROUND

Medication errors commonly occur as the patient moves through the continuum of care. According to the Joint Commission, 63% of reported medication errors were due to a breakdown in communication which could have been avoided by completing a medication reconciliation.[1] In 2004, the Joint Commission included medication reconciliation across the continuum of care to the 2005 National Patient Safety Goal #8. Thus, medication reconciliation can and should occur at each care transition. This includes when the patient is moving from one healthcare setting to another, transferring from one level of care to another (e.g., intensive care unit to medical unit), and seeing different care providers.

Medication reconciliation is defined as the process of creating the best possible medication list of all the medications the patient should be taking, which is accomplished by comparing the patient's active medication orders or prescriptions to all of the medications that the patient has been taking.[1,2] The goal of medication reconciliation is to avoid medication errors that may lead to an unwanted adverse drug event. Medication errors commonly occur when there are medication discrepancies in the patient's medication list(s). These errors may consist of omissions, commissions, dosing errors, duplications, or drug interactions.[1,3]

There are many strategies to facilitate a successful medication reconciliation. These strategies include but are not limited to focusing on high-risk patient groups, especially if limited resources are an issue.[3] These high-risk patient groups include but are not limited to those with evidence of polypharmacy, use of high-risk medications (anticoagulants, insulin, etc.), limited health literacy, elderly, complex medical or behavioral conditions, and medical conditions or procedures that fall under the Centers for Medicare & Medicaid Services Hospital Readmissions Reduction Program (acute myocardial infarction, chronic obstructive pulmonary disease, heart failure, pneumonia, coronary artery bypass graft surgery, and elective primary total hip arthroplasty and/or total knee arthroplasty).

Additionally, when implementing medication reconciliation, one should consider utilizing all pharmacy personnel to perform various aspects of the medication reconciliation process. Pharmacy technicians and student pharmacists may collect a medication history and pharmacy residents and licensed pharmacists can complete the medication reconciliation process. Furthermore, it is important to obtain buy-in from leadership and frontline staff to help champion the medication reconciliation program. Lastly, engage the patient and empower them to take charge in ensuring they are receiving and taking the best possible medication list.

Completing medication reconciliation is not without its challenges. Medication reconciliation may be difficult to implement due to patient, provider, and healthcare setting barriers.[3] Patients may have low health literacy and have limited knowledge of their medications. Providers may have limited time to complete the medication reconciliation or have limited knowledge of what medication(s) the patient is taking if it was prescribed by a different provider. Furthermore, healthcare setting factors such as limited resources (staff, technology, etc.) may not allow for successful medication reconciliation.

The facilitators and barriers to a successful medication reconciliation discussed above should be considered prior to implementing a medication reconciliation program. Once ready to conduct a medication reconciliation for a patient, the process should be approached in a stepwise fashion. The stepwise approach to medication reconciliation as defined by the Joint Commission and the Institute for Healthcare Improvement is listed in Table 2-1.

At the end of the medication reconciliation process, there should be an accurate, up-to-date best-possible medication list that should include all prescription drugs, over-the-counter medications, vitamins, minerals, herbals, and other supplements. The best-possible medication list should also include topical products, inhalers, injectables, eye- and ear-drops, and nose sprays that are often left off mistakenly by patients during medication history and review.

TABLE 2-1.   Medication Reconciliation Approach

Joint Commission[1]	Institute for Healthcare Improvement[2]
1. Develop a list of current medications	1. Verification (collection of the medication history)
2. Develop a list of medications to be prescribed	2. Clarification (ensuring that the medications and doses are appropriate)
3. Compare the medications on the two lists	3. Reconciliation (documentation of changes in the orders)
4. Make clinical decisions based on the comparison	
5. Communicate the new list to appropriate caregivers and to the patient	

The medication reconciliation process for each healthcare setting may vary slightly, but the ultimate goal is to get the patient their correct medications and make decisions based off of the comprehensive list at all transition points. To learn more about the medication process in the inpatient and outpatient setting, please refer to the cases in the "Transitions of Care at Hospital Discharge" and the "Transitions of Care in the Outpatient Setting" chapters in this book.

PATIENT PRESENTATION

Chief Complaint

"My right hip hurts and nothing is helping."

History of Present Illness

KR is a 76-year-old male who was admitted to the hospital for total hip arthroplasty (THA) after a long history of left hip pain due to osteoarthritis. He had been suffering with progressively worse pain in the left hip over the past few years and has tried analgesics with minimal pain relief. KR has experienced increased difficulty with performing activities of daily living and can no longer tolerate the pain. He now opts for surgical intervention. KR successfully underwent left THA with no complications. He is now post-op day 3 and is ready for discharge back to the assisted living facility with outpatient physical therapy.

Past Medical History

Diabetes
Early-onset dementia
Glaucoma
Gout
Heart failure with preserved ejection fraction
Hyperlipidemia
Hypertension
Osteoarthritis

Surgical History

N/A

Family History

Father: died at age 75 from natural causes
Mother: died at age 67 from heart attack

Social History

Widowed; one grown son lives out of state.

Immunization

Up to date

Insurance

Medicare and Medicaid

Allergies

No known allergies

Prior-to-Admission Medications

- Allopurinol 100 mg, 1 tablet PO once daily
- Amlodipine 10 mg, 1 tablet PO once daily
- Calcium carbonate/vitamin D 600 mg/800 IU, 1 tablet PO once daily
- Capsaicin 0.025% cream, apply thin film topically to left hip 3 to 4 times daily
- Celecoxib 100 mg, 1 capsule PO twice daily
- Furosemide 20 mg, 1 tablet PO daily as needed for edema
- Latanoprost 0.005%, 1 drop in each eye once daily in the evening
- Lisinopril 10 mg, 1 tablet PO once daily
- Metformin 1000 mg, 1 tablet PO twice daily
- Multivitamin, 1 tablet PO once daily
- Rosuvastatin 20 mg, 1 tablet PO daily

Current Medications

- Acetaminophen 325 mg, 1–2 tablets PO every 4–6 hours PRN for mild-moderate pain
- Atorvastatin 40 mg, 1 tablet PO daily
- Heparin 5000 units subcutaneously every 8 hours
- Hydrocodone/acetaminophen 5/500 mg, 1 tablet PO every 4–6 hours PRN for severe pain
- Regular insulin sliding scale
- Latanoprost 0.005%, 1 drop in each eye once daily in the evening
- Omeprazole 20 mg, 1 capsule PO daily

Physical Examination

▸ *Vital Signs*

Temp 98.7°F (37.1°C), P 82, RR 18, BP 146/82 mmHg, O_2 saturation 99%

▸ *General*

Comfortable other than left hip pain.

▸ *HEENT*

PERRLA, EOMI.

▸ *Respiratory*

Normal breath sounds.

▸ *Cardiovascular*

Normal rate and regular rhythm.

▸ *Abdominal*

Soft. Bowel sounds are normal. No abdominal tenderness.

▸ *Neurologic*

Alert and oriented to person, place, and time.

▸ *Musculoskeletal*

Normal other than decreased range of movement in external rotation of left hip.

▸ *Extremities*

Skin is warm and dry. Not edematous.

Findings

Na = 138 mEq/L	Hgb = 12 g/dL
K = 6 mEq/L	Hct = 36.8%
Cl = 100 mEq/L	Plt = 156 × 10³/uL
CO_2 = 25 mEq/L	WBC = 6.2 × 10³/uL
BUN = 13 mg/dL	
SCr = 0.66 mg/dL	
Glu = 200 mg/dL	

Imaging Studies

Left hip radiograph shows severe osteoarthritis with marked loss of joint cartilage and osteophytes.

QUESTIONS

1. When should medication reconciliation occur for KR?
   A. Admission to the assisted living facility
   B. Admission to the hospital
   C. Discharge from the hospital
   D. All of the above

2. When asking the patient or caregiver questions to elicit a best-possible medication history, which of the following questions are phrased most appropriately?
   A. Do you take lisinopril at home?
   B. Do you take lisinopril for your high blood pressure?
   C. What medications do you take at home for your high blood pressure?
   D. What medications do you take for your hypertension?

3. Which of the following actions are most appropriate for completing a medication reconciliation for KR?
   A. Contact the assisted living facility to determine the list of medications the patient is currently taking prior to hospital admission
   B. Interview the patient to determine the list of medications they are currently taking prior to hospital admission
   C. Obtain the medication list that is being ordered during the hospital stay
   D. A and C

4. When reconciling the prior-to-admission medication list to the current hospital medication list, what unintentional error of omission did you identify?
   A. Acetaminophen was started in the hospital
   B. Amlodipine was not restarted in the hospital
   C. Latanoprost was started in the hospital
   D. Lisinopril was not restarted in the hospital

5. When reconciling the prior-to-admission medication list to the current hospital medication list, what unintentional error of commission did you identify?
   A. Atorvastatin was started in the hospital
   B. Hydrocodone/acetaminophen was started in the hospital
   C. Calcium carbonate/vitamin D was not restarted in the hospital
   D. Omeprazole was started in the hospital

6. Which of the following discrepancies between the prior-to-admission medication list and the inpatient medication orders is intentional and does not require immediate intervention during the hospital stay?
   A. Capsaicin was not restarted
   B. Insulin regular was started
   C. Rosuvastatin was not restarted
   D. All of the above

7. You noticed that allopurinol was not restarted in the hospital. What do you do?
   A. Contact the hospital team and recommend that they restart home dose of allopurinol
   B. Contact the hospital team and tell them it is appropriate to hold allopurinol during the hospital stay but should resume allopurinol at discharge
   C. Tell the patient we will discontinue allopurinol permanently since he is not experiencing any gout symptoms

D. Tell the patient we will hold allopurinol during the hospital stay since he is not experiencing any gout symptoms

8. KR was started on rivaroxaban prior to discharge for the prevention of postoperative venous thromboembolism. Which of the following statement(s) is an appropriate counseling point?

A. Heparin was given to you in the hospital to thin your blood to prevent clots from forming. At the assisted living facility, you will take rivaroxaban tablets instead of injectable heparin.

B. Rivaroxaban can increase your risk of bleeding. Talk to your doctor if you are experiencing any signs or symptoms of bleeding.

C. Talk to your doctor before you take over-the-counter medications such as aspirin or NSAIDs (ibuprofen, naproxen) because those medications can also increase your risk of bleeding.

D. All of the above.

9. Now that the patient is transferred back to the assisted living facility, at a minimum, how often must a pharmacist perform a drug regimen review for this patient?

A. Daily

B. Weekly

C. Once per month

D. Twice per month

REFERENCES

1. Joint Commission. Using medication reconciliation to prevent errors. Available at www.jointcommission.org/assets/1/18/SeA_35.pdf. Accessed January 25, 2006.

2. Institute for Healthcare Improvement. Prevent Adverse Drug Events by Implementing Medication Reconciliation. Available at http://www.ihi.org/resources/Pages/Tools/HowtoGuidePreventAdverseDrugEvents.aspx. Last updated December 2011.

3. Sponsler KC, Neal EB, Kripalani S. Improving medication safety during hospital-based transitions of care. *Cleve Clin J Med.* 2015;82(6):351-360.

4. Xarelto (rivaroxaban) [package insert]. Titusville, NJ: Janssen Pharmaceutical Companies; 2020.

5. The Lewin Group. CMS Review of Current Standards of Practice for Long-Term Care Pharmacy Services. Available at https://www.cms.gov/Research-Statistics-Data-and-Systems/Statistics-Trends-and-Reports/Reports/downloads/lewingroup.pdf. Accessed December 30, 2004.

3 Transitions of Care at Hospital Discharge

Laressa Bethishou   Kristen Herzik

BACKGROUND

As patients navigate through the healthcare system, there is both a need and an opportunity to support safe and effective transitions of care. The potential for complications such as medication errors and adverse events arise as patients transition from one care setting to another. Poor communication between healthcare providers, lack of standardized processes, and discrepancies in electronic health records contribute to ineffective care transitions. However, this is especially problematic when discharging from hospital to another care setting, which can lead to unwanted outcomes including medication errors and hospital readmissions.[1,2]

In 2012, the Center for Medicare & Medicaid Services (CMS) implemented the Hospital Readmission Reduction Program (HRRP), which penalizes hospitals for excessive readmissions. Hospitals receive a reduction in payment for all-cause readmission within 30 days for patients with applicable conditions, including pneumonia, heart failure, myocardial infarction, chronic obstructive pulmonary disease, and hip or knee arthroplasty.[3] As a result, healthcare institutions have an invested interest to improve transitions of care in an effort to reduce hospital readmissions and improve healthcare outcomes.

Transitions of care at hospital discharge requires a multidisciplinary effort and involves bridging the gap between inpatient and other care environments. The pharmacist can play a valuable role in supporting patients during transitions of care. Contributions include comprehensive discharge planning, medication reconciliation, discharge education, addressing access barriers, and care coordination to ensure appropriate follow-up and monitoring. A pharmacist providing transitions of care services in the hospital setting must have knowledge and training in how to navigate both the inpatient and outpatient healthcare environments to effectively provide these services to their patients.

Comprehensive discharge planning should begin early on in admission to anticipate and address barriers to discharge.

A collaborative interprofessional approach should incorporate the unique needs of each patient in creating and implementing a plan and appropriate follow-up. Patient-specific needs may vary based on their discharge disposition, level of independence and caregiver support, functional and cognitive capacity, and financial resources. For example, identifying a patient started on a known expensive brand name medication or one that is known to carry outpatient formulary restrictions allows time to triage and address those issues prior to discharge to ensure medication therapy is not interrupted. As healthcare providers reconcile medications, provide education, and support continuity of care, they should consider what support the patient requires to safely transition to their next care setting.

Medications should be reconciled at the time of admission, during transfers, and upon hospital discharge.[4] An accurate best-possible medication history (BPMH) which identifies medications the patient was taking prior to admission is imperative for patient safety as well as to limit unnecessary interruption in medication therapy during hospitalization. It also ensures a smoother discharge and prevents medication errors.[5] Discharge medication reconciliation involves comparing the medications taken prior to admission, those taken during the hospital stay, and the discharge medication list. Discharge medication reconciliation should identify and resolve discrepancies, including inappropriate prescribing, incorrect dosing, drug interactions, adherence barriers to ensure the list is safe, follows guideline-directed medication therapy, and is cost effective for the patient. If issues are identified, they should be resolved prior to discharge.

Once the discharge medication list is complete, pharmacists can provide discharge medication education. This comprehensive education reviews the entire medication list, including new medications, changes to existing medications, and discontinued medications. Education should address discussion of adverse effects, correct administration, and relevant disease state counseling. If an educational deficit is contributing to poor adherence, this can be addressed as well. Discharge counseling should incorporate open-ended questions and teach-back to assess patient understanding. If there are co-learners, or the need for an interpreter, discharge counseling may need to be scheduled in advance to ensure all appropriate caregivers are present.

The pharmacist can also improve medication access by identifying and resolving barriers to medication use. Patient-specific factors such as health and functional status, cultural factors and personal beliefs, health literacy, and socioeconomic status should be assessed as possible barriers which can impact access to medications and healthcare services. Pharmacists can support patients by securing access to medications and durable medical equipment (DME) by ensuring prescriptions are accurate and have refills, checking stock at outpatient pharmacies, and coordinating home or bedside delivery. Patients requiring DME, such as diabetes supplies or nebulizers, may require support and education in securing and learning how to use their equipment. Pharmacists can also assist patients with financial barriers such as recommending a cheaper alternative regimen, or assistance with initiating prior authorizations or identifying additional support to supplement payment such as manufacturer coupons or drug discount programs. Pharmacists can also provide follow-up and monitoring instructions, which supports continuity of care beyond hospital discharge.

The pharmacist can support patients by working closely with the healthcare team to provide continuity of care services and ensure the coordination of appropriate follow-up and monitoring to optimize medication management. Confirming that appointments with outpatient providers are made, pertinent labs will be drawn, or ensuring adequate support for medication-related needs, such as coordination with home health for administration of IV medications, are some ways pharmacists can assist in supporting discharge needs. Continuity of care services that the pharmacist can provide directly to the patient, patient representative, or caregiver may include a post-discharge follow-up by means of a phone call.[6] Post-discharge follow-up calls are recommended to occur within 72 hours to promote early detection of adverse events that may lead to a hospital readmission. The calls may also occur at additional intervals depending upon readmission risk assessment of the patient.

In collaboration with the patient and their healthcare team, the pharmacist can support safe and effective transitions of care at hospital discharge. While pharmacist interventions may vary depending on the healthcare institution and patient-specific needs, comprehensive discharge planning should incorporate these interventions to support continuity of care at hospital discharge.

PATIENT PRESENTATION

Chief Complaint

Confusion

History of Present Illness and Hospital Course

JS is an 85-year-old female with a past medical history of hypertension, hypothyroidism, and osteoporosis who presented to the emergency department yesterday with confusion secondary to a suspected urinary tract infection. She also complains of difficulty sleeping, dizziness, and that she has been more forgetful lately and has had difficulty managing her medications. Her confusion has now resolved, and she is ready for discharge.

Past Medical History

Hypertension
Hypothyroidism
Osteoporosis

Social History

The patient is widowed and lives alone, but her daughter visits her regularly.

She does not smoke but drinks 1 to 2 glasses of brandy every evening to help her relax.

She does not have much of an appetite, eating 3 small meals per day.

Immunization

Up to date

Insurance

Aetna Medicare Complete

Allergies

Penicillin (hives)

Home Medications

- Alendronate 70 mg PO weekly
- Amlodipine 10 mg PO daily
- Calcium 1000 mg PO daily
- Metoprolol tartrate 25 mg PO bid
- Synthroid 88 mcg PO daily

Inpatient Medications

- Calcium 1000 mg PO daily
- Levofloxacin 500 mg PO daily
- Levothyroxine 88 mcg PO daily
- Metoprolol tartrate 25 mg PO bid

Physical Examination

▶ **HEENT**

PERRLA, denies vertigo, congestion, sore throat, chills, lightheadedness.

▶ **Cardiovascular**

Denies racing heart, orthopnea. No edema.

▶ **Respiratory**

No wheezing, cough, or hemoptysis.

▶ **Gastrointestinal**

No abdominal pain, constipation, diarrhea, or change in frequency.

▶ **Urinary**

No hematuria or urgency.

▶ **Cardiovascular**

Regular rate and rhythm,

▶ **Musculoskeletal**

Gait not assessed.

▶ **Neurologic**

Confusion has resolved.

▶ **Psychological**

Denies depression, anxiety, or change in mood.

▶ **Vital Signs (on discharge)**

Temp 98.7°F, P 68 bpm, RR 16, BP 105/65 mmHg, Ht: 70″, Wt: 65 kg

Values (on discharge)

Na = 133 mEq/L
K = 3.6 mEq/L
Glucose = 98 mg/dL
Creatinine = 1.0 mg/dL
BUN = 19 mg/dL
AST = 21 U/L
ALT = 23 U/L
WBC = 6.1×10^3/uL
Hemoglobin = 13 g/dL
Hematocrit = 37 g/dL

Imaging/Diagnostic

U/A normal.

QUESTIONS

1. What additional information provided by the patient is important to consider in transitioning her from hospital to home?
   A. "I take some over-the-counter medications to help with sleep"
   B. "I have difficulty moving around my house and sometimes stumble"
   C. "My daughter helps me fill my pill box each week"
   D. All of the above

2. The patient informs us she also takes a few over-the-counter medications. In her purse, we find the following:
   Excedrin Migraine
   St. John's Wort
   Tylenol PM
   ZZZQuil Nighttime Sleep-Aid
   Which is the most appropriate action to optimize her medication management?
   A. Continue all of her over-the-counter medications as they are safe
   B. Discontinue her St. John's Wort as it may be contributing to her confusion
   C. Discontinue her Excedrin Migraine as caffeine may be affecting her sleep
   D. Discontinue only one of her sleep-aid medications as this is a duplication of therapy

3. What should be included in comprehensive discharge planning for our patient?
   A. A referral to physical and occupational therapy
   B. Ensuring coverage and appropriate prescribing for new medications only
   C. Asking the patient's daughter to reach out to home health services
   D. All of the above

4. The physician has ordered the following discharge medications for JS:
   Alendronate 70 mg PO weekly
   Amlodipine 10 mg daily
   Metoprolol tartrate 25 mg PO bid
   Synthroid 88 mcg PO daily
   Calcium 1000 mg PO daily
   Which of the following interventions is most appropriate for our patient?
   A. Her medication list is appropriate and does not require any interventions
   B. Her levofloxacin should be continued as the patient requires one additional dose
   C. Her amlodipine should be held due to her low blood pressure today
   D. The patient should be discharged on levothyroxine 88 mcg daily

5. Which of the following statements regarding discharge education is correct?
   A. Medication education should review her new medications only
   B. The patient should be engaged using open-ended questions and the teach-back method
   C. The patient, her daughter, and an interpreter should be present
   D. All of the above

6. When providing discharge education, which of the following counseling points is most appropriate for this patient?
   A. It is okay to continue drinking alcohol as there are no adverse effects or medication interactions

B. Separate administration of calcium and metoprolol tartrate by at least 2 hours
C. Take alendronate at the same time as calcium for optimal benefit
D. Incorporate sleep hygiene to help improve mental and physical health

7. Which of the following should be monitored and followed up with post discharge?
A. Blood pressure
B. Depression
C. Symptoms on admission (dizziness, confusion, trouble sleeping)
D. All of the above

REFERENCES

1. Joint Commission. Transitions of Care: The Need for a More Effective Approach to Continuing Patient Care. Hot Topics in Health Care. Available at https://www.jointcommission.org/-/media/deprecated-unorganized/imported-assets/tjc/system-folders/topics-library/hot_topics_transitions_of_carepdf.pdf?db=web&hash=CEFB254D5EC36E4FFE30ABB20A5550E0.

2. Wong JD, Bajcar JM, Wong GG, et al. Medication reconciliation at hospital discharge: evaluating discrepancies. *Ann Pharmacother.* 2008;42(10):1373-1379.

3. Centers for Medicare and Medicaid Services. Hospital Readmission Reduction Program. Available at https://www.cms.gov/Medicare/Medicare-Fee-for-Service-Payment/AcuteInpatientPPS/Readmissions-Reduction-Program. Baltimore MD.

4. Agency for Healthcare Research and Quality. Medication Reconciliation. Available at https://psnet.ahrq.gov/primer/medication-reconciliation. Rockville, MD.

5. Murphy EM, Oxencis CJ, Klauck JA, et al. Medication reconciliation at an academic medical center: implementation of a comprehensive program from admission to discharge. *Am J Health Syst Pharm.* 2009;66:2126-2131.

6. Bethishou L, Herzik K, Fang N, Abdo C, Tomaszewski DM. The impact of the pharmacist on continuity of care during transitions of care: a systematic review. *J Am Pharm Assoc (2003).* 2020;60(1):163-177.e2.

4 Transitions of Care in the Outpatient Setting

Jessica Wooster

BACKGROUND

Pharmacist involvement in transitional care management activities post-discharge is critical to ensure safe and effective medication therapy outcomes in patients as they move between healthcare settings. Pharmacists in the outpatient setting, including both community and ambulatory care, may be involved prior to discharge in patient care activities such as medication reconciliation prior to discharge, bedside teaching of discharge medications, patient assistance for improving medication access, or prescription delivery services such as "meds-to-beds." Post-discharge, outpatient pharmacists may conduct follow-up phone calls to patients preferably made within 1 to 3 days once the patient returns home. The purpose of these calls is to reinforce any patient education, ensure the patient has received their medications, check on the clinical status of the patient, and to answer any questions they may have. In addition, this is a good time to ensure the patient has a post-discharge follow-up appointment scheduled with a primary care or specialty physician to ensure continuity of care. The next point of contact differs in purpose and timing based on location.

Community pharmacists often see patients post-discharge before any other healthcare team members. This is because patients and/or caregivers head to the community pharmacy shortly after hospital discharge to pick up prescriptions. This represents a great opportunity for the community pharmacist to perform medication reconciliation with the patient's discharge prescriptions and the prior-to-admission medication list. If any medication errors or discrepancies are identified, the pharmacist should hold off on dispensing these prescriptions, inform the patient of the situation, and call the prescribing physician to resolve the issue. This patient encounter is also a good time to reinforce patient education on medications, conditions, and self-care. We can also answer any questions or address concerns the patient may have now that they have left the hospital. Community pharmacists often have an established rapport with patients, which may result in the patient feeling at ease to ask questions and follow pharmacist recommendations on medication adherence and self-care.

Ambulatory care pharmacists are able to interact with patients at their post-discharge follow-up appointments that should occur within 1 to 2 weeks based on patient medical complexity. It is important for patients to attend these clinic appointments as this is often where adverse events can be mitigated and ultimately prevent unplanned emergency department visits or hospitalizations. At the clinic, pharmacists may be involved in the following transitions of care activities: post-discharge phone calls or communication, review of discharge information, medication reconciliation, follow-up on pending labs or diagnostic tests, optimization of medication therapy, providing patient education, and addressing patient-specific needs or barriers to care.

Medication reconciliation should occur at every transition of care for a patient. At the clinic setting, it can be helpful to have patients bring in their medication bottles, their medication list, and conduct a patient interview on what the patient is taking and how they are taking it. It is important to have this best-possible medication list and an accurate idea of patient adherence to medications before clinical decisions can be made at the appointment. If any medication errors or discrepancies are identified, these can be resolved at the clinic visit. In addition to ensuring medications prescribed are safe, it is just as important to optimize a patient's medications to promote better health outcomes.

Once a therapy plan is devised between the physician, pharmacist, and patient and/or caregiver, the pharmacist can implement the plan by providing thorough education on the new medications prescribed, also noting any medication changes or discontinued medications the patient is to be aware of. The clinic setting is a good time to reinforce patient education on medications, conditions, and self-care that was previously covered at hospital discharge. At this time, it is appropriate to address additional concerns or expand upon topics such as smoking cessation, healthy eating, and physical activity. We should also seek to identify and address patient-specific barriers such as medication access issues, low health literacy, and adherence problems, along with any other issues that may require attention. Collaborating with healthcare team members both within and across healthcare settings to provide effective patient handoffs, share accurate patient health information, and resolve discrepancies will promote optimal health outcomes across the continuum of care.

PATIENT PRESENTATION

Chief Complaint

"I need something to help my heartburn."

History of Present Illness

MW is a 42-year-old male presenting with his wife to the pharmacy for some advice. His wife has noticed over the past week he seems to be clearing his throat frequently and has not slept well at night. MW complains he awakens in the middle of the night about 3 or 4 nights a week with a burning feeling in his chest and throat, and he prefers to sleep in the recliner chair. This in turn has worsened his back pain, requiring him to take Tylenol more frequently. His wife is worried these symptoms are related to his heart. MW denies difficulty swallowing, painful swallowing, and weight loss. He has been trying Pepcid for these heartburn symptoms, but it has not been helping.

Past Medical History

Hypertension
Hyperlipidemia
Heartburn
Back pain

Family History

Father died of heart attack at 57 yo
Mother died of cancer at 72 yo

Social History

Denies smoking, drinking, and illicit drug use

Immunization History

Up to date

Insurance

Medicare

Allergies

Sulfa medications

Home Medications

Amlodipine	10 mg	1 tablet by mouth daily
Simvastatin	40 mg	1 tablet by mouth daily at bedtime
Tylenol	325 mg	1 tablet by mouth every 4 to 6 hours as needed for pain
Pepcid	20 mg	1 tablet by mouth as needed for heartburn
Aspirin	81 mg	1 tablet by mouth daily

Physical Examination

▶ *Vital Signs*

Temp 98.4, P 64, RR 16, BP 122/82 mmHg, Ht: 5 ′11″, Wt: 175 lbs

▶ *General*

Patient appears well nourished and in no apparent distress.

QUESTIONS

1. When treating a patient in a community pharmacy, it is important to collect enough information in order to appropriately assess their problem(s). MW presents to the pharmacy with many GERD symptoms. Which of the following signs/symptoms are NOT suggestive of GERD?
   A. Frequent clearing of throat
   B. Night-time burning sensations
   C. Sleeps with head elevated in a recliner
   D. Back pain

2. Collecting a thorough medical history and pertinent information on the patient's current complaint is critical so you can determine if they are able to be treated or must be referred to a physician for further evaluation. Often a patient approaches the community pharmacist for a product recommendation, but the pharmacist must gather sufficient information to determine if they are excluded from self-care.

   Which of the following is an alarm symptom that would warrant the pharmacist to advise the patient to follow up with their physician for further evaluation?
   A. Painful swallowing
   B. Regurgitation
   C. Nighttime awakenings
   D. Water brash

3. It is important to take a thorough medication history, including nonprescription agents, in all patients who visit the outpatient community pharmacy for advice, whether they are in the pharmacy system or not. Once we obtain an accurate medication history, we can assess for any medication-related problems.

   When interviewing the patient to obtain a medication history, you realize that one of MW's medications may worsen symptoms of GERD. Which medication can worsen MW's GERD?
   A. Tylenol
   B. Simvastatin
   C. Amlodipine
   D. Pepcid

4. Once we collect patient information, assess their current problem(s), and determine we can treat the patient, we can then begin to develop and implement a therapy plan. This plan may include both pharmacologic and nonpharmacologic therapies.

   Which of the following nonpharmacological steps for MW will help alleviate his GERD symptoms?

A. Eating foods that exacerbate heartburn to increase tolerance
B. Eating large meals three times a day
C. Eating a snack immediately before bedtime to help settle the stomach.
D. Avoidance of meals 2 to 3 hours before bedtime

5. Once we determine if we are able to treat the patient, we may develop and implement a therapy plan including both pharmacologic and nonpharmacologic therapies. In the community pharmacy, we may recommend over-the-counter (OTC) medications without a prescription as appropriate based on the patient's problem(s). If prescription agents must be recommended, it is dependent upon state law and collaborative practice agreements in place to determine if the community pharmacist may provide a prescription or if a physician referral is warranted.

   What OTC treatment approach is the best for the patient at this time?
   A. Recommend omeprazole, a proton pump inhibitor (PPI) for a 2-week trial
   B. Recommend use of antacids such as Tums as needed
   C. Recommend lifestyle changes
   D. Referral to physician

6. After therapy plan implementation, it is important for the patient to follow up at regular intervals to ensure their symptoms are improving and not worsening, and to address any questions or concerns. In the community pharmacy, this can be done via phone call to the patient, or when they come back to the pharmacy to pick up their prescriptions.

   Two weeks later, MW returns to the pharmacy for a follow-up recommendation after he runs out of his OTC medication you recommended. He states the medication helped reduce his heartburn symptoms, but the symptoms returned when he ran out the medication. He has been incorporating all of the lifestyle changes you recommended, but it is not sufficient to resolve his symptoms. What is the best recommendation at this time?
   A. Recommend omeprazole, a proton pump inhibitor (PPI)
   B. Recommend cimetidine, a histamine-2 receptor antagonist (H2RA)
   C. Recommend use of antacids such as Tums as needed
   D. Refer to physician

7. In the ambulatory care pharmacy setting, whether having a medication list in their chart or not, it is important to conduct a thorough medication history and reconciliation at every visit. Which of the following should be used to conduct a medication reconciliation?
   A. Medication list in the electronic health record (EHR)
   B. Patient interview to assess adherence
   C. Contact the patient's community pharmacy
   D. All of the above

8. When the physician asked MW what he has tried in the past for his GERD symptoms, he could not recall. He remembers that he tried another medicine before the omeprazole but does not remember the name. Which of the following is the best step to obtain an appropriate medication history?
   A. Read all of the names of OTC heartburn therapies and let the patient guess
   B. Call the community pharmacy so they may check his medication profile
   C. Assume it was another PPI and pick one to put in record
   D. Assume it was an H2RA and pick one to put in patient record

9. Pharmacist-provided education on medication changes, importance of adherence, and adverse effects is a key component to ensure optimal patient outcomes during transitions of care. Patient-centered education helps the patient take an active role in their treatment and informs them of adverse effects to watch for and precautions that may warrant self-care or a call to the pharmacist or physician.

   MW presents to a follow-up visit at his primary care physician's office. He informs the physician he ordered omeprazole 20 mg online and it has been working well to reduce his heartburn symptoms. He says he only has symptoms when he eats very acidic foods such as tomato sauce, which he tries to avoid. He takes omeprazole 20 mg in the morning before breakfast daily. He is concerned that PPI use may be harmful, as his daughter told him he should discontinue it because it may lead to adverse health outcomes. Which of the following is a risk associated with long-term PPI use?
   A. Community-acquired pneumonia
   B. *Clostridium difficile* risk factor
   C. Asthma
   D. Osteopenia

REFERENCES

1. Katz PO, Gerson LB, Vela MF. Guidelines for the diagnosis and management of gastroesophageal reflux disease. *Am J Gastroenterol.* 2013;108(3):308-328.
2. Omeprazole [package insert]. Wilmington, DE: AstraZeneca Pharmaceuticals LP; revised 2016.

Section 2

Therapy Adherence and Patient Care Barriers

The Importance of Addressing Financial Barriers

Jessica Wooster   Laressa Bethishou

BACKGROUND

Identifying and addressing financial barriers is an important intervention which can facilitate safe and effective transitions of care. When optimizing medication therapy, pharmacist interventions should include addressing cost. This may include initiating prior authorizations, selecting cheaper alternatives when available, or identifying resources to supplement the cost of medications. When available, collaboration with case management and social work can be valuable in meeting the unique and individual needs of the patient.

PATIENT PRESENTATION

Chief Complaint

"My chest hurts bad. It felt like heartburn at first, now it's a stabbing pain!"

History of Present Illness

JJ, a 43-year-old African American male with a medical history of hypertension, is admitted to the coronary care unit with chest pain. He reports the pain started this morning at work and felt like bad heartburn. Over the next few hours, it progressed to a sharp, shooting pain that is 8 out of 10 on a severity pain scale. He chewed four baby aspirin tablets with no relief, but he recalled you were to take aspirin if you think you are having a heart attack. When asked about adherence, he reports taking his medication only when his blood pressure is high, which he believes is indicated by a headache. He also says this way his prescription lasts much longer. Patient states he does not have a blood pressure monitor at home. Patient often forgets his cholesterol medication at bedtime as he often falls asleep on the couch after a few beers.

Past Medical History

Hypertension, hyperlipidemia

Family History

Both parents with hypertension and coronary artery disease (CAD)

Social History

High school janitor. On his feet all day at work but limited physical activity outside of work.

Smokes one pack per day × 20 years, denies illicit drug use. He lives alone.

Drinks 2 to 3 beers in the evenings and on weekends.

Diet consists of fast food, eats at a local diner, and microwave meals.

Insurance

Medicaid

Immunization

Up to date

Allergies

No known drug allergies

Home Medications

- Amlodipine 10 mg PO daily
- Simvastatin 20 mg daily at bedtime
- Aleve 220 mg PRN pain/headache
- Aspirin 81 mg PRN pain

Physical Examination

▶ *Vital Signs*

Temp 98.6°F, P 110, RR 22, BP 170/98 mmHg, pO_2 98%, Ht: 5'10", Wt: 129 kg

▶ *General*

Anxious, disheveled, overweight male in distress.

▶ *HEENT*

PERRLA, EOMI.

▶ *Pulmonary*

No wheezing, crackles, rales; increased respirations.

▶ *Cardiovascular*

Normal heart sounds, no murmurs, rubs, or gallops.

▶ *Abdomen*

Non-distended, nontender, normal bowel sounds.

▶ *Genitourinary*

Normal male genitalia, no complaints of dysuria or hematuria.

▶ *Neurologic*

Alert and oriented × 4.

▶ *Extremities*

No edema, peripheral pulses intact, normal ROM.

Values

Na = 132 mEq/L
K = 4.0 mEq/L
Cl = 102 mEq/L
CO_2 = 22 mEq/L
BUN = 15 mg/dL
SCr = 1.0 mg/dL
Glu = 132 mg/dL
Hgb = 14.9 g/dL
Hct = 40%
Plt = 115 × 10^3/mm³
WBC = 2 × 10^3/mm³
Troponin I = 8.6 ng/ mL
Total CK = 86 ng/mL
NT pro-BNP = 400 pg/mL
Ca = 9.7 mg/dL
Mg = 2 mg/dL
AST = 22 IU/L
ALT = 30 IU/L
T Bili = 1.6 mg/dL
Alk Phos = 75 IU/L
PO_4 = 2.4 mg/dL
Albumin = 3.5

Fasting Lipids

Total Cholesterol = 240 mg/dL
LDL-C = 140 mg/dL
HDL-C = 34 mg/dL
Trig = 188 mg/dL

Diagnostic Tests

▶ *Electogcardiogram*

HR 112 bpm, ST-segment elevation in leads II, III, and a VF consistent with acute inferior myocardial infarction (MI).

Emergency Department Summary

In the ED, an ECG showed ST-segment elevation and they administered morphine, oxygen, IV unfractionated heparin (UFH), IV nitroglycerin, and oral metoprolol. A stat cardiologist consultation was requested, and now JJ is on his way to the cardiac catheterization lab for percutaneous coronary intervention (PCI).

▶ *Cardiac Catheterization*

70% proximal stenosis in the RCA with thrombus; drug-eluting stent (DES) implanted. Patient loaded with ticagrelor 180 mg, UFH continued, and eptifibatide infusion was started.

Note: Patient reached cath lab within 1 hour of ED arrival.

▶ *Echocardiogram*

LVEF of 65%

Discharge Summary

Patient is stable and no longer complaining of pain, just states he is tired and ready to go home. Patient is ready to be discharged later today which is 3 days post-MI. The discharge nurse brings JJ's discharge paperwork for him to sign, and hands him his prescriptions to be filled. He says to the nurse "These medications better be cheap, I only have about $40 to spare each month and it is usually spent on beer."

QUESTIONS

1. Which risk factors need to be modified to reduce the patient's risk of readmission?
   A. Nonadherence and financial barriers
   B. Poor diet and lifestyle
   C. NSAID use
   D. Smoking
   E. All of the above

2. Which of the following nonadherence barriers must be addressed in the outpatient setting to ensure this patient remains compliant to all medications?
   A. Cost of medications
   B. Forgetfulness
   C. Transportation issues
   D. Lack of perceived benefit

3. How do you plan to address this patient's adherence issues?
   A. Tailor medication education and self-care to patient's health literacy level
   B. Employ motivational interviewing techniques
   C. Tell him to download phone application to help him remember to take his medications

D. Assist JJ with figuring out how he can afford his medications

E. Recommend physician to change to medications taken once daily when possible

4. Which of the following dual antiplatelet therapies and duration is recommended after an acute myocardial infarction?

A. Prasugrel for a minimum of 6 months and aspirin indefinitely

B. Prasugrel and aspirin for a minimum of 12 months

C. Clopidogrel for minimum of 6 months and aspirin indefinitely

D. Ticagrelor for minimum of 12 months and aspirin indefinitely

5. What other medications do you want to ensure JJ is prescribed at discharge?

A. Evidenced based beta blocker

B. ACEi/ARB

C. Nitroglycerin SL

D. High intensity statin

E. All of the above

6. Which of the following referrals are recommended to ensure continuity of care and improved outcomes?

A. Cardiovascular rehabilitation program

B. Community pharmacist to administer pneumococcal vaccine

C. Pain management

D. Home healthcare

7. JJ arrives at the community pharmacy to pick up his discharge prescriptions. They are all ready, except for the antiplatelet medication, as it is out of stock. The pharmacist anticipates it will come in tomorrow and she will call him when it is ready. The next day, the pharmacist calls JJ to let him know the prescription is ready but informs him it will cost $360, and that is with a discount coupon she found. He informs her he cannot afford the medication, so the community pharmacist says she will call the doctor to see what to do next. As it is a Friday, she informs JJ it may not be until Monday before she hears back from the doctor's office. Sunday in the middle of the night JJ awakens to a sharp pain across his chest. This pain is familiar and he fears the worst, so he calls 911. He arrives at the ED and it is confirmed he has occluded his stent and is having a heart attack.

Which of the following actions may have prevented JJ's hospital readmission?

A. Early request for prior authorization of ticagrelor

B. Motivational interviewing to assess adherence

C. Send antiplatelet prescription to another pharmacy that has it in stock

D. Assist with transportation services to pick up his medications

8. Which of the following transitional care management activities may have identified JJ's risk of readmission?

A. Follow-up phone call within 48 hours post-discharge to determine JJ had not received his antiplatelet medication

B. Post-discharge appointment 7 to 14 days at the cardiology clinic

C. Medication reconciliation prior to hospital discharge

D. Bedside education on medications prior to hospital discharge.

REFERENCES

1. Amsterdam EA, Wenger NK, Brindis RG, et al. 2014 AHA/ACC guideline for the management of patients with non–ST-elevation acute coronary syndromes: a report of the American College of Cardiology/American Heart Association Task Force on Practice Guidelines. *J Am Coll Cardiol.* 2014;23;64(24):e139-e228.

2. Levine GN, Bates ER, Bittl JA, et al. 2016 ACC/AHA guideline focused update on duration of dual antiplatelet therapy in patients with coronary artery disease: a report of the American College of Cardiology/American Heart Association Task Force on Clinical Practice Guidelines. *J Am Coll Cardiol.* 2016;68(10):1082-1115.

6 Communication and Health Literacy

Roxane L. Took

BACKGROUND

A well-known barrier in transitions of care is clear, consistent communication. This applies to both communication among the healthcare team and communication with patients. The Joint Commission estimates approximately 80% of serious medical errors are caused by poor communication between healthcare providers.[1] Ineffective communication has been shown to lead to fragmented care and patient dissatisfaction.[2]

Several resources are available to improve communication between healthcare providers. The Joint Commission's Targeted Solutions Tool (TST) for Hand-Off Communications can be used to identify barriers to exceptional performance and provide specific solutions to address each barrier. The Joint Commission recommends using the mnemonic SHARE to address causes of unsuccessful hand-offs: **S**tandardizing critical content, **H**ardwiring within your system by using standardized forms, tools, and methods, **A**llow opportunity for others to ask questions and clarify information obtained, **R**einforce quality and measurement through accountability and monitoring, and **E**ducate and coach staff using standardized training on how to conduct successful hand-offs.[3] Another standardized communication method is the SBAR (situation, background, assessment, and recommendation) technique. Although the SBAR technique was originally created by the U.S. Navy for communication on nuclear submarines, it has been highly utilized by the healthcare system as a template to provide clear communication. Using this method, healthcare providers are encouraged to first describe the situation and then provide succinct yet thorough background that may be needed. In the final steps, an assessment and clear recommendation should be communicated to the next provider.[4]

The use of standardized forms during transfers between various levels of care has demonstrated improved communication of patients' advanced directives, improved safety perceptions, and increased patient satisfaction and outcomes.[5-7] The development of a standardized hand-off tool with a coordinated medication reconciliation increases patient satisfaction regarding medication knowledge and meeting health-related goals, especially when patients are able to speak to a pharmacist about their medications.[8]

In addition to providing clear communication to the healthcare team, it is important to ensure that information is appropriately communicated to the patient. Proper training on health literacy should be implemented to teach the healthcare team how to measure health literacy and to provide strategies to break down difficult concepts. Resources available to help assess health literacy and train staff include the Agency for Healthcare Research and Quality (AHRQ) Pharmacy Health Literacy Center, Health Literacy Tool Shed, and the AHRQ Health Literacy Universal Precautions Toolkit. Patients at high risk for low health literacy should be screened. One popular tool that can be used to assess health literacy is the Newest Vital Sign (NVS). According to the 2003 National Assessment of Adult Literacy, individuals at high risk for poor health literacy are patients who are male, Hispanic, Black, American Indian/Alaska native, English language learners, older than 65 years of age, living below poverty level, and did not receive their high school diploma.[9]

PATIENT PRESENTATION

Chief Complaint

Follow-up visit after recent 3-day hospitalization. Patient was discharged 10 days ago.

History of Present Illness

Stephen is a 51-year-old African American male who presented to the emergency department 13 days ago with an elevated blood pressure reading of 182/96 mmHg (manual). His community pharmacist called 911 because each of his automated blood pressure readings on the grocery store blood pressure kiosk were greater than 140/90 mmHg, and these readings were elevating steadily over a period of 15 minutes. The patient stated that he experienced chest tightness and anxiety but had no signs or symptoms of shortness of breath, chest pain, or visual changes at the time he was admitted to the emergency department. He was transferred to the cardiac care unit for approximately 2 days for monitoring before being discharged to home. When discharged from the hospital he was told to discontinue his losartan and start Edarbi® (azilsartan). He was also told to monitor his blood pressure once daily. Today he presents to the family medicine clinic for a follow-up visit for this recent hospitalization. Patient seems disheveled and states he cannot find his hospital information and blood pressure readings. He fears that this paperwork may have been misplaced.

Past Medical History

Anxiety × 4 months
Depression × 4 months
Dyslipidemia (DLD) × 5 years
Hypertension (HTN) × 2 years
Obesity (unknown duration)

Surgical History

Appendectomy (22 years ago)

Family History

Both parents are still living
Father: 81 y/o, has DLD, HTN, and type 2 diabetes (DM)
Mother: 74 y/o, has DLD, HTN, and hypothyroidism
Brother died at age 17 from a motor vehicle collision; no other siblings

Social History

Full-time bakery worker at a local grocery store.
Divorced; lives with his two daughters who attend a nearby high school.
Highest level of education: some high school.
Does not engage in routine exercise.
Denies tobacco and illicit drug use.
Drinks alcohol 1 to 2 times per year for special occasions.
Drinks 1 to 2 cups of coffee per day (190 mg of caffeine).

Immunization

Up to date

Insurance

Receives commercial insurance benefits through his employer.

Allergies/Intolerances

ACE-I—induced cough from lisinopril

Home Medications

- Alprazolam 0.25 mg PO tid PRN
- Atorvastatin 40 mg PO daily
- Azilsartan (Edarbi) 40 mg PO daily
- Citalopram 20 mg PO daily
- Men's multivitamin PO daily

Physical Examination

▸ Vital Signs

Temp 97.4°F, RR 16 bpm, HR 80 bpm, BP: 140/82 mmHg (left arm, manual); 144/86 mmHg (right arm, manual), O_2 sat: 98% (room air), Ht: 5′7″, Wt: 202 lbs, BMI: 31.3 kg/m²
   Newest vital sign score: 3

▸ General

Awake, alert, and oriented. No acute distress. Well-developed, and well-nourished.

▸ Skin

Warm, dry, and intact without rashes or lesions. Nail beds pink with no cyanosis or clubbing.

▸ HEENT

Normocephalic; PERRLA, EOMI, mucous membranes are moist.

▸ Neck

Supple, nontender, without lymphadenopathy, masses, or thyromegaly.

▸ Pulmonary

Clear to auscultation and percussion without rales, rhonchi, wheezing, or diminished breath sounds.

▸ Cardiovascular

RRR without murmurs, gallops, or rubs.

▸ Abdomen

Soft, non-distended, nontender, normal bowel sounds; normal male genitalia.

▸ Genitourinary

No back or flank tenderness; no complaints of dysuria or hematuria.

▸ Neurologic

A&O × 3; CN II—XII intact; DTRs 2+; patient irritable.

▸ Extremities

Full range of motion noted in all joints. Muscle strength is 5/5 bilaterally. Tendon function normal. Pulses palpable. Steady gait noted.

Values

Na = 140 mEq/L
K = 3.9 mEq/L

Cl = 107 mEq/L
CO_2 = 28 mmol/L
BUN = 22 mg/dL
SCr = 1.1 mg/dL
Glu = 89 mg/dL
Ca = 8.9 mg/dL
Mg = 2.1 mEq/L
Phos = 2.7 mg/dL
AST = 15 U/L
ALT = 12 U/L
T Bili = 0.9 mg/dL
Alk Phos = 52 IU/L

Refill History (from the Community Pharmacy)

Outpatient medication history confirmed with community pharmacist as per the list below. Patient states that he takes his alprazolam as needed for anxiety. He was taking the citalopram as needed but found that it did not help as much as alprazolam, so he discontinued this medication. Prior to his hospitalization, he was taking his losartan and hydrochlorothiazide as needed when he felt like his blood pressure was getting high. He was told by the hospital to discontinue his losartan and start azilsartan. He states that he had difficulty paying for his medications prior to starting azilsartan; he states he cannot afford to continue this azilsartan. Prior to starting azilsartan he admits to delaying medication refills because he was waiting for his next paycheck to help pay for his medications. He expresses that he is overwhelmed with the number of medications that he is taking and their cost. Stephen is the sole provider for his home, and although he has insurance benefits through his employer he still struggles to pay for his medications, especially around prom/homecoming season and the holidays.

Drug	Day Supply	Pick-up Date	Amount Paid
Azilsartan (Edarbi) 40 mg	30	10 days ago	$20
Alprazolam 0.25 mg	30	25 days ago	$1.25
Alprazolam 0.25 mg	30	55 days ago	$1.25
Losartan 100 mg	30	63 days ago	$4
Citalopram 20 mg	30	63 days ago	$4
Alprazolam 0.25 mg	30	85 days ago	$1.25
Hydrochlorothiazide 12.5 mg	30	215 days ago	$4
Alprazolam 0.25 mg	30	215 days ago	$1.25
Losartan 50 mg	30	127 days ago	$4
Hydrochlorothiazide 12.5 mg	30	127 days ago	$4
Citalopram 20 mg	30	127 days ago	$4

QUESTIONS

1. What critical information could have been shared with the patient's primary care provider to prevent initial hospitalization?
   A. Lack of access to a home blood pressure monitor
   B. Other home medications (herbals, vitamins, supplements)
   C. Refill history and barriers to adherence
   D. The patient's alcohol and caffeine use

2. Which of the following is the most appropriate strategy hospitals can utilize to provide more effective transitions of care?
   A. Each nurse should create their own communication template to allow for customization
   B. Obtain medication history exclusively from the patient to avoid confusion and misinformation from other sources
   C. Provide standardized training to staff on how to conduct successful hand-off
   D. When communicating with other healthcare providers, encourage the use of abbreviations during healthcare provider communications to decrease word count

3. Which correctly identifies the purpose of the SBAR technique?
   A. To assess clinical health status
   B. To estimate the risk of medication non-adherence
   C. To identify baseline health literacy
   D. To provide clear communication

4. When communicating with other healthcare providers using the SBAR tool, which of the following statements can be categorized as situation (S)?
   A. I'm calling about Stephen Hill, date of birth: 5/18/1969. He presents to the clinic today for a follow-up visit after a recent hospitalization.
   B. I recommend that we continue citalopram.
   C. The patient has a history of anxiety, depression, dyslipidemia, hypertension, and obesity.
   D. The patient is not experiencing any signs or symptoms of anxiety or depression.

5. Which are identified barriers to optimizing Stephen's health?
   A. Health literacy and cost
   B. Health literacy and side effects
   C. Side effects and transportation
   D. Transportation and cost

6. The suitability assessment of materials (SAM) instrument can be used to identify an appropriate blood pressure handout for this patient. According to this instrument, which content should be included in the handout to help increase readability?
   A. A detailed image to show how blood is pumped throughout the body.
   B. A summary to retell key messages.
   C. Information provided at an eighth grade reading level.
   D. Size 12 font with no bolding or colors

7. What is the most appropriate way to communicate medication changes to this patient?
   A. Do not provide explanation to the patient, it will only overwhelm him. Send all new electronic prescriptions to the pharmacy.
   B. Provide brief verbal directions regarding medication changes to the patient.
   C. Provide verbal and written directions regarding medication changes to the patient along with a medication list.
   D. Talk to the patient about all the medication options that are available, explain why those options were ruled out, and then provide a detailed explanation about all medication changes

8. Upon reflection of this case, what information should have been communicated upon discharge and to whom?
   A. Discharge paperwork to the patient's healthcare providers
   B. Family history of hypertension with community pharmacist
   C. Patient's medical insurance to the community pharmacy
   D. Patient's medication list to a family member

REFERENCES

1. Joint Commission on Accreditation of Healthcare Organizations. Joint Commission Center for Transforming Healthcare. Hand-Off Communications. Available at http://www.centerfortransforminghealthcare.org/projects/detail.aspx?Project=1.
2. Mansukhani RP, Bridgeman MB, Candelario D, Eckert LJ. Exploring transitional care: evidence-based strategies for improving provider communication and reducing readmissions. *P T*. 2015;40(10):690-694.
3. Joint Commission Center for Transforming Healthcare Releases Targeted Solutions Tool for Hand-Off Communications. Available at https://www.jointcommission. org/-/media/deprecated-unorganized/imported-assets/tjc/system-folders/blogs/tst_hoc_persp_08_12pdf.pdf?db=web&hash=BA7C8CDB4910EF6633F013D0BC08CB1C#:~:text=Ineffective%20hand%2Doff%20communication%20is,during%20the%20transfer%20of%20patients.
4. Heinrichs WM, Bauman E, Dev P. SBAR "flattens the hierarchy" among caregivers. *Stud Health Technol Inform*. 2012;173:175-182.
5. Zafirau WJ, Snyder SS, Hazelett SE, Bansal A, McMahon S. Improving transitions: efficacy of a transfer form to communicate patients' wishes. *Am J Med Qual*. 2012;27(4):291-296.
6. Alimenti D, Buydos S, Cunliffe L, Hunt A. Improving perceptions of patient safety through standardizing handoffs from the emergency department to the inpatient setting: a systematic review. *J Am Acad Nurse Pract*. 2019;31(6):354-363.
7. Nakayama DK, Lester SS, Rich DR, et al. Quality improvement and patient care checklists in intrahospital transfers involving pediatric surgery patients. *J Pediatr Surg*. 2012;47(1):112-118.
8. Vuong V, O'Donnel D, Navare H, et al. BOOMR: Better Coordinated Cross-Sectoral Medication Reconciliation for Residential Care. *Healthc Q*. 2017;20:34-39.
9. Kutner M, Greenberg E, Jin Y, et al. The health literacy of America's adults: results from the 2003 National Assessment of Adult Literacy (NCES 2006–483). U.S. Department of Education. Washington, DC: National Center for Education Statistics. 2006.
10. SAM. Suitability Assessment of Materials for Evaluation of Health-Related Information for Adults. Available at http://aspiruslibrary.org/literacy/SAM.pdf.
11. Johnson A, Sandford J. Written and verbal information versus verbal information only for patients being discharged from acute hospital settings to home: systematic review. *Health Educ Res*. 2005;20(4):423-429.
12. Hersh L, Salzman B, Snyderman D. Health literacy in primary care practice. *Am Fam Physician*. 2015;92(2):118-124.

7 ¿Hablas Espanol?: Language Discordance in Transitions of Care

Danielle M. Candelario   Khyati Patel

BACKGROUND

Transition from hospital to home is a particularly difficult stage in the care transitions continuum due to the likelihood of breakdowns in communication between providers and patients alike. Patients of ethnically diverse backgrounds are particularly vulnerable to breakdowns in the transition process due to language and cultural discordance, posing a significant challenge to the provision of quality healthcare.[1,2]

Language barriers contribute to health disparities among patients with limited English proficiency. Language discordant care between patients and their providers increases the risk for a variety of poor outcomes.[3-7] The identification and resolution of this particular barrier can improve medication adherence, health education, patient satisfaction, and patient–provider relationships.

PATIENT PRESENTATION

Chief Complaint

Admitted for total knee arthroplasty (TKA)

History of Present Illness

Mariana is a 72-year-old female with a 3-year history of degenerative joint disease of the right knee with a profound exacerbation of her symptoms 2 months prior to admission. She was admitted 3 days ago for a TKA, which proceeded unremarkably. Postoperatively, she has been managed for VTE prophylaxis with enoxaparin and an intermittent pneumatic compression device. Her pain is well controlled with oxycodone via patient-controlled anesthesia (PCA) pump. Mild confusion noted on postoperative day 1 has mostly been resolved. She has a multi-year history of well-controlled hypertension and epilepsy, hypercholesterolemia of unknown duration, and chronic kidney disease (CKD) for the last 7 years. Based on the medication list, the patient was asked about coronary artery disease but she denies any history of heart disease. All history is per daughter translating at the bedside.

Past Medical History

Hypertension
Hypercholesterolemia
CKD Stage G3b
Epilepsy

Surgical History

Hysterectomy (unknown year)
Right TKA (3 days prior)

Family History

She is adopted and is not familiar with birth parents' medical history

Social History

Relocated to the US 3 years ago from Ecuador. Speaks minimal English — preferred language is Spanish.
Married with two adult children; lives with spouse.
Denies alcohol, tobacco, or recreational/illicit drug use.

Immunization

Up to date

Insurance

Medicaid

Allergies

No known drug allergies

Home Medications

- Hydrochlorothiazide 25 mg PO once daily
- Losartan 50 mg PO once daily
- Aspirin 81 mg PO once daily

- Atorvastatin 40 mg PO once daily
- Phenytoin 100 mg PO twice daily

Physical Examination

▶ Vital Signs

Temp 98.7°F, P 72, RR 16, BP 110/68 mmHg, pO$_2$ 96% RA, Ht 5′3″, Wt 96 kg, Pain 4/10

▶ General

The patient is a well-developed, well-nourished elderly female who is oriented to time, place, and person but intermittently mildly confused to time.

▶ Skin

Warm and dry; no rashes.

▶ HEENT

Normocephalic; PERRLA, EOMI; normal sclerae; mucous membranes are moist; TMs intact; oropharynx clear.

▶ Neck/Lymph Nodes

Supple, (−) for lymphadenopathy.

▶ Lungs

Normal breath sounds.

▶ Cardiovascular

RRR without murmur; normal S1 and S2.

▶ Abdomen

Soft, NT/ND; (+) bowel sounds; no organomegaly.

▶ Genitourinary

No back or flank tenderness; normal female genitalia.

▶ Extremities

1 to 2+ swelling around the right knee. Incision over the anterior aspect of the right knee with diffuse mild soft tissue swelling.

▶ Neurologic

A&O × 3; CN II—XII intact; DTRs 2+; normal mood and affect.

Laboratory Values (on discharge day)

Na = 138 mEq/L
K = 4.0 mEq/L
Cl = 99 mEq/L
CO2 = 26 mEq/L
Scr = 1.5 mg/dL
BUN = 20 mg/dL
Glu = 103 mg/dL
AST = 24 IU/L
ALT = 22 IU/L

T Bili = 0.9 mg/dL
Hgb = 14 g/dL
Hct = 39 %
Plt = 232 × 10³/μL
WBC = 7.8 × 10/mm³

Discharge Information

72-year-old Hispanic female s/p right TKA ready for discharge to home.

The patient had an unremarkable postoperative recovery with some mild confusion which has since resolved. At the time of discharge, she is moderately independent with regard to all of her functions, including dressing, bathing, toileting, transfers, and she can ambulate with a walker. Currently she reports 4/10 pain. She is discharged with instructions to increase her strength, endurance, and knee range of motion with visiting physical therapy and wound management three times per week. Safety issues are to be addressed with the patient on an ongoing basis. Patient will require a rolling walker for discharge. She is to follow up with her surgeon in 1 week. Daughter is not present for discharge education; patient denied an interpreter and will be sent home with discharge paperwork. Husband to pick up the patient for 5 pm discharge.

QUESTIONS

1. What would be the most optimal pain control strategy for Mariana upon discharge?
   A. Continue oxycodone PCA pump
   B. Convert oxycodone PCA pump to celecoxib 200 mg PO daily
   C. Convert oxycodone PCA pump to oxycodone/APAP 7.5 mg/325 mg PO q4−6h PRN
   D. Convert oxycodone PCA pump to tramadol 50 mg PO q4−6h PRN

2. What VTE prophylaxis agent is the most appropriate for Mariana post discharge?
   A. Apixaban 2.5 mg PO twice daily
   B. Dabigatran 150 mg PO once daily
   C. Enoxaparin 30 mg SQ q12h
   D. Enoxaparin 100 mg SQ q12h

3. Which of the following is the most appropriate decision regarding her aspirin use?
   A. Change aspirin to clopidogrel 75 mg PO once daily
   B. Continue aspirin 81 mg PO once daily
   C. Discontinue aspirin 81 mg PO once daily
   D. Increase aspirin to 325 mg PO once daily

4. Which of the following is most likely to be a barrier to an effective transition to home for Mariana?
   A. Chronic kidney disease
   B. Lack of transportation home
   C. Lack of private healthcare insurance
   D. Misunderstanding of discharge instructions

5. Which of the following communication techniques may help identify a language discordance between the patient and the providers?
   A. Active listening
   B. Nonverbal communication interpretation
   C. Teach-back method
   D. Motivational interviewing

6. Which of the following services is mandated by federal regulatory agencies for Mariana?
   A. Confirmation of receipt of discharge paperwork
   B. Offer to counsel on new medications
   C. Language assistance
   D. Seventy-two-hour discharge follow-up

7. After confirming that Mariana requires language assistance, which of the following would be the most appropriate action:
   A. Provide printed materials in Spanish
   B. Request the assistance of a hospital employee who speaks the appropriate language
   C. Require the presence of a family member to provide translation
   D. Utilize medical translator mobile application

8. Which of the following is a best practice for utilizing a medical interpreter?
   A. Seat the interpreter next to or slightly behind the patient
   B. Speak directly to the interpreter
   C. Speak slowly to allow for simultaneous translation
   D. Utilize "tell him/her" statements to assist interpreter

9. Which of the following needs to be done to ensure timely receipt of prescription medications for an 8 pm administration?
   A. Arrange for home delivery with a social worker
   B. Call outpatient pharmacy to ensure stock and hours of operation
   C. Fax prescription to mail order pharmacy
   D. Hold discharge for the next morning to provide night-time dose

REFERENCES

1. Rayan N, Admi H, Shadmi E. Transitions from hospital to community care: the role of patient-provider language concordance. *Isr J Health Policy Res.* 2014;3:1-8.
2. Jowsey T, Gillespie J, Aspin C. Effective communication is crucial to self-management: the experiences of immigrants to Australia living with diabetes. *Chronic Illn.* 2011;7:6-19.
3. Fernandez A, Schillinger D, Warton EM, et al. Language barriers, physician-patient language concordance, and glycemic control among insured Latinos with diabetes: the Diabetes Study of Northern California (DISTANCE). *J Gen Intern Med.* 2011;26(2):170-176.
4. Detz A, Mangione CM, Nunez de Jaimes F, et al. Language concordance, interpersonal care, and diabetes self-care in rural Latino patients. *J Gen Intern Med.* 2014;29:1650-1656.
5. Traylor AH, Schmittdiel JA, Uratsu CS, et al. Adherence to cardiovascular disease medications: does patient-provider race/ethnicity and language concordance matter? *J Gen Intern Med.* 2010;25(11):1172-1177.
6. Ngo-Metzger Q, Sorkin DH, Phillips RS, et al. Providing high-quality care for limited English proficient patients: the importance of language concordance and interpreter use. *J Gen Intern Med.* 2007;22:324-230.
7. Carrasquillo O, Orav EJ, Brennan TA, et al. Impact of language barriers on patient satisfaction in an emergency department. *J Gen Intern Med.* 1999;14(2):82-87.
8. Falck-Ytter Y, Francis CW, Johanson NA, et al. Prevention of VTE in orthopedic surgery patients. *Chest.* 2012;141:e278S-e325S.
9. Lexicomp online. Hudson, Ohio: Wolters Kluwer Clinical Drug Information, Inc.; 2020; June 13, 2020.
10. US Preventive Services Task Force. Aspirin Use to Prevent Cardiovascular Disease and Colorectal Cancer: Preventative Medication. https://www.uspreventiveservicestaskforce.org/uspstf/recommendation/aspirin-to-prevent-cardiovascular-disease-and-cancer. Rockville, MD. 2016.
11. American Community Survey Reports: English-Speaking Ability of the Foreign-Born Population in the United States: 2012. https://www2.census.gov/library/publications/2014/acs/acs-26.pdf. Washington, DC. 2014.
12. Schillinger D, Piette J, Grumbach K, et al. Closing the loop: physician communication with diabetic patients who have low health literacy. *Arch Intern Med.* 2003;163:83-90.
13. Agency for Healthcare Research and Quality: Making Healthcare Safer III: A Critical Analysis of Existing and Emerging Patient Safety Practices. Available at https://www.ahrq.gov/sites/default/files/wysiwyg/research/findings/making-healthcare-safer/mhs3/making-healthcare-safer-III.pdf. Rockville, MD. 2020.
14. Tamura-Lis W. Teach-Back for quality education and patient safety. *Urol Nurs.* 2013;33:267-271.
15. Ha Dinh TT, Bonner A, Clark R, et al. The effectiveness of the teach-back method on adherence and self-management in health education for people with chronic disease: a systematic review. *JBI Database System Rev Implement Rep.* 2016;14(1):210-247.
16. Jucket G, Unger K. Appropriate use of medical interpreters. *Am Fam Physician.* 2014;90:476-480.
17. Health and Human Services Department: Nondiscrimination in Health Programs and Activities. A Rule by the Health and Human Services Department on 05/18/2016. https://www.federalregister.gov/documents/2016/05/18/2016-11458/nondiscrimination-in-health-programs-and-activities. Washington, DC. 2016.

18. Centers for Medicare & Medicaid Services. TOOLKIT for Making Written Material Clear and Effective SECTION 5: Detailed guidelines for translation PART 11 Understanding and using the "Toolkit Guidelines for Culturally Appropriate Translation". Available at https://www.cms.gov/Outreach-and-Education/Outreach/WrittenMaterialsToolkit/Downloads/ToolkitPart11.pdf. Washington, DC. 2010.

19. National Council on Interpreting in Health Care: FAQ – Translators and Interpreters. https://www.ncihc.org/faq-for-translators-and-interpreters#:~:text=A%20qualified%20interpreter%20is%20an,Ethics%20and%20Standards%20of%20Practice. Washington, DC.

8 Addressing Patient Nonadherence

Amulya Uppala

BACKGROUND

Medication adherence is defined as the degree to which the patient's behavior corresponds with the agreed-upon recommendation from a healthcare provider. According to the World Health Organization (WHO), in developed countries only 50% of patients who have chronic diseases such as hypertension and diabetes adhere to treatment recommendations.[1] Thus, nonadherence roughly accounts for 100,000 preventable deaths and $100 billion in preventable medical costs annually.[2] Due to rising healthcare costs and poor health outcomes, it is important to educate healthcare professionals about barriers, measurements, and strategies to improve medication adherence.

Potential barriers to medication adherence can be categorized as either patient related or treatment related. Patient-related barriers include lack of motivation, depression, denial, cognitive impairment, substance or alcohol abuse, cultural or alternate beliefs, and low healthcare literacy. Treatment-related barriers may include complex treatment regimens, actual or concern for potential side effects, inconvenience, cost of medications, and time management. Other important barriers to adherence include poor provider–patient relationship, inadequate follow-up, suboptimal discharge planning, and treatment of an asymptomatic disease (i.e., hypertension, HIV, diabetes).[2,3] Healthcare professionals who have a heightened awareness of these barriers and predictors to nonadherence can effectively target successful interventions. It is important to understand that age, race, sex, and socioeconomic status have not been consistently associated as major predictors for nonadherence; they should not be the sole basis for decisions when evaluating interventions to improve adherence.[2]

There are many direct and indirect methods to measure adherence. Multiple methods of measuring adherence should be used since there is no gold standard, and each method has potential advantages and disadvantages. Direct methods such as observing medication administration and drug levels are objective, but they can be impractical or impossible to do depending on the patient and the drug administered.

Thus, indirect methods such as patient self-reporting, patient questionnaire, pill-counting prescription bottles, monitoring prescription refills, and measuring clinical response (i.e., heart rate, blood pressure, temperature) should be used for most patients. Many of these indirect methods are simple and easy to perform, but the disadvantages include patient distortion of the data, susceptibility of error in polypharmacy, and lack of direct correlation between the method and the clinical response. During patient interview, it is important to understand that patients often do not want to disappoint their providers and may not be forthcoming. Thus, asking questions in a nonjudgmental and non-confrontational manner makes most patients feel comfortable and facilitates an open conversation.[2]

Numerous interventions are available to improve medication adherence. The most common methods include patient education about medications and disease states, improved communication between healthcare professional and patient, increasing accessibility to care via more clinic hours or frequent appointments, and improving dosing schedules.[2] Patient education about medications and disease states are helpful to improve health literacy, decrease concerns about medication side effects, motivate patients on self-care, and increase awareness of the harmful effects of asymptomatic diseases.[1] One of the most effective ways to improve dosing schedules is by simplifying medication regimens from multiple times a day to once daily or transdermal applications; simplifying dosing frequencies has been correlated with increased adherence rates.[4] Medication reminders such as pill boxes, pill cards, compliance packaging, or technology integration can be employed based on patient preference. Pill boxes come in various forms where patients can easily organize their medications for the week based on the time of the day. Pill cards are small pocket cards that contain name, dose, indication, instructions for morning, afternoon, evening, and nightly doses. Compliance packaging is when pills are prepackaged by an outside vendor into unit doses based on the time of the day. Technological methods include automatic text messages or smartphone free medication adherence applications.[5] Increasing accessibility to care and improving patient–provider relationships can encourage patients to be accountable for adherence and decrease healthcare-associated barriers to adherence.

Finally, at the end of every patient appointment, phone call, or patient education healthcare providers should employ the teach-back technique to ensure adequate understanding of the information. One study estimates that patients do not remember or misinterpret 50% of information given by providers. When using teach-back, use open-ended questions to discuss information (i.e., tell me in your own words how to take this medication). Most importantly, avoid quizzing the patient, using medical jargon or highly technical terms, appearing rushed or annoyed, and simple yes or no questions.[6]

PATIENT PRESENTATION

Chief Complaint

"I have too many medications and sometimes I forget to take them."

History of Present Illness

AN is a 55-year-old Caucasian male who presents for his transitions of care medication management appointment 1 week after being discharged from the hospital. This was the second time he was hospitalized in the past 2 months. He was admitted for uncontrolled hypertension (HTN) and chest pain; however, his cardiac workup was negative. He was treated for high blood pressure prior to being discharged.

Past Medical History

Asthma
HTN
Type 2 diabetes (T2DM)
Coronary artery disease (CAD) with one stent 2 months ago

Surgical History

None

Family History

Father: has HTN and diabetes.
Mother: had diabetes and HTN; died from a heart attack 4 years ago.

Social History

He is divorced and has one son and one daughter.
He lives alone and works as an overnight truck driver. He also indicates he sometimes works as an Uber driver to earn extra cash.
He does not smoke or do illicit drugs but has a history of doing recreational drugs during high school.
He did not attend college.
He drinks socially but no more than 1 to 2 drinks a week.

Immunization

Up to date

Insurance

United Health Care. He also a prescription insurance plan with OptumRx

Allergies

No known drug allergies

Home Medications (per electronic medication record)

- Fluticasone-Salmeterol 250/50 mcg 1 puff bid and as needed q6h for shortness of breath
- Aspirin 81 mg PO qam
- Prasugrel 10 mg PO qam
- Atorvastatin 40 mg PO nightly
- Metoprolol tartrate 50 mg PO bid
- Furosemide 40 mg PO qam
- Lisinopril 10 mg PO bid
- Clonidine 0.1 mg PO tid
- Hydrochlorothiazide 25 mg PO qam
- Metformin IR 1000 mg PO bid

Pertinent Laboratory Findings (from 1 month ago)

▶ *BMP*

Na = 140 mEq/L
Cl = 100 mmol/dL
K = 3.4 mEq/L
BUN = 16 mg/dL
SCr = 0.6 mg/dL
HCO = 25 mmol/L
Glu = 100 mg/dL
Mg = 2.0 mg/dL
Ca = 8.2 mg/dL
HbA1c = 7.0 %

▶ *Lipid Panel*

Total Cholesterol: 190 mg/dL
HDL: 41 mg/dL
LDL: 112 mg/dL
TG: 150 mg/dL

▶ *Thyroid function*

TSH: 1.9

QUESTIONS

1. Prior to the patient's visit, you are reviewing his chart to evaluate potential reasons for nonadherence. Which one

of the below is the most likely treatment-related barrier to medication adherence for AN?

A. Cost of medications
B. Complexity of treatment
C. Low educational level
D. Lack of motivation

2. Which of the following is an optimal way to measure adherence in this patient?

A. Having the patient fill out a simple questionnaire about adherence
B. Conducting a "brown bag" medication review and pill count
C. Contacting the pharmacy to get his prescription fill record
D. All of the above

3. Which of the following questions is appropriate to ask when assessing the patient for adherence?

A. I know it must be difficult to take all your medications regularly. How often do you miss taking them?
B. Do you not take your medications as prescribed?
C. When you feel like your blood pressure is under control, do you sometimes stop taking your medicine?
D. A and C

4. After interviewing the patient, the following clarified medication list was obtained:

Fluticasone-Salmeterol 250/50 mcg 1 puff bid and as needed q6h PRN for SOB

Aspirin 81 mg PO qam

Prasugrel 10 mg PO qam

Atorvastatin 40 mg PO am

Lisinopril 10 mg PO once to twice daily

Hydrochlorothiazide 25 mg PO qam

Metformin 1000 mg PO once to twice daily (depends on if he remembers the second dose)

His vitals in the office include BP 145/95 mmHg, HR 88 bpm, Temp 98.6°F, blood glucose 110.

Upon further discussion he admits that he does not take the metoprolol because it makes him tired, he stopped taking the furosemide because he couldn't sleep due to the constant need to wake up to urinate. He never took the clonidine because it is too many times a day to remember. He also admits he is on the road often, so he just forgets to take his evening doses of most of his medications. Overall, he is frustrated because he doesn't understand why he needs to take "so many medications."

Which criteria are major predictors for poor adherence in our patient?

A. Treatment of asymptomatic disease, side effects of medication, lack of insight into illness, age
B. Age, socioeconomic status, race, lack of insight into treatment, complexity of treatment
C. Treatment of asymptomatic disease, side effects of medication, lack of insight into illness, complexity of regimen

D. Race, poor provider–patient relationship, side effects of medication, lack of insight into illness

5. Which if the following methods is the most effective strategy to improve medication adherence for AN?

A. Change the lisinopril from 10 mg twice daily to 20 mg once daily
B. Add a clonidine patch to the current regimen
C. Change metformin to glipizide 2.5 mg twice daily
D. Discontinue the aspirin

6. Which of the following adherence aids will be the helpful for AN?

A. A pill card for his wallet and refrigerator
B. A pill box
C. An electronic medication reminder application
D. All of the above

7. Which of the following questions is the most optimal method to provide teach-back for AN?

A. In order to prevent hypertensive urgency, it is important to take your medications on time. How will you take your medications at home?
B. I understand we reviewed a lot of information. Just to review when you get home, how many pills will you take? What time will you take them?
C. I know I gave you a lot of new information. Do you have any questions?
D. We spent a lot of time reviewing and modifying your medications. Can you quickly tell me the changes we made?

REFERENCES

1. World Health Organization. Adherence to long-term therapies: evidence for action. Available at http://www.who.int/chp/knowledge/publications/adherence_report/en/. Accessed June 7, 2020.
2. Osterberg L, Blaschke T. Adherence to medication. *N Engl J Med.* 2005;353(5):487-497.
3. Kleinsinger F. The unmet challenge of medication nonadherence. *Perm J.* 2018;22:18-33.
4. Claxton AJ, Cramer J, Pierce C. A systematic review of the associations between dose regimens and medication compliance. *Clin Ther.* 2001;23:1296-1310.
5. American Association of Colleges of Pharmacy and National Community Pharmacist Association. Medication adherence educators toolkit. Available at https://www.aacp.org/sites/default/files/aacp_ncpa_medication_adherence_educators_toolkit_0.pdf. Accessed June 7, 2020.
6. U.S. Department of Health and Human Services, Agency for Healthcare Research and Quality. Use the teach-back method: Tool #5. February 2015. Available at http://www.ahrq.gov/professionals/quality-patient-safety/quality-resources/tools/literacy-toolkit/healthlittoolkit2-tool5.html. Accessed June 7, 2020.

9 Trucking Along: Medication Adherence with Provider Issues

Takova D. Wallace-Gay   Rachel A. Bratteli

PATIENT PRESENTATION

Chief Complaint

"My ankles are swollen, and I can hardly do anything without getting short of breath."

History of Present Illness

JW is a 51-year-old African American male presenting to the pharmacy-led heart failure clinic for 1-month follow-up of a heart failure with reduced ejection fraction (HFrEF) exacerbation that required hospitalization. It has been 6 months since his last office visit since he works as a truck driver and has been out of town. He asks for a prescription for compression socks as he has noticed increased swelling in his ankles.

Patient states he has been out of his furosemide and carvedilol for the past month. The carvedilol was added after his last hospital discharge. When asked about why he has not filled these, he states he does not like the side effects of the furosemide and often misses the second dose of carvedilol. He begrudgingly has a cell phone for his work but does not like to use technology. He states adherence to his other medications, though he sometimes makes it to the pharmacy a couple of days late due to his work. His primary care physician told him at discharge, "If you do not get it together and take your medications, you are going to die."

Past Medical History

Hypertension (HTN)
HFrEF
Hyperlipidemia (HLD)
Myocardial infarction (MI) (status post CABG)
History of illicit drug use

Surgical History

CABG (3 years ago)

Family History

Mother: died age 60 from MI
Father: died age 51 from MI
Siblings: three brothers, one brother deceased from MI; three sisters, two of whom have had at least one MI before age 60
All siblings have HTN

Social History

Divorced and lives alone; monogamous female partner frequently visits.
Truck driver for the past 30 years (self-insured).
(+) Tobacco—1½ pack per day × 25 years.
(+) Alcohol—1 to 2 beers daily.

Immunization

Up to date

Insurance

Medicaid

Allergies

No known drug allergies

Home Medications

- Aspirin 81 mg PO qd
- Atorvastatin 80 mg one-half tablet PO qd
- Furosemide 40 mg PO bid
- Potassium 20 mEq PO qd
- Lisinopril 20 mg PO qd
- Carvedilol 12.5 mg PO bid
- NTG 0.4 mg SL, PRN chest pain
- Acetaminophen 500 mg PO, PRN back pain

Physical Examination

▶ *Vital Signs*

Temp 98.6°F, P 68 bpm, RR 18 breaths/minute, BP 167/80 mmHg, pO2 97%, Ht: 5'11", Wt: 160 lbs, BMI: 22.31 kg/m²

▶ *General*

Well developed, well-nourished male in no acute distress.

▶ *HEENT*

PERRLA, EOMI.

▶ *Pulmonary*

(+) SOB.
(+) Bilateral crackles.

▶ *Cardiovascular*

NSR, no m/r/g.

▶ *Abdomen*

Soft, non-distended, nontender, (+) bowel sounds.

▶ *Genitourinary*

Normal male genitalia; denies abnormal discharge.

▶ *Neurologic*

(+) Headaches 1−2 times a week, A&O × 3.

▶ *Extremities*

2−3+ bilateral LEE.

Laboratory Findings

Na = 136 mEq/L	Hgb = 15.2 g/dL	Ca = 8.5 mg/dL
K = 4.8 mEq/L	Hct = 39.3%	Mg = 2.1 mEq/L
Cl = 98 mEq/L	Plt = 256 × 10³/mm³	Phos = 3.5 mg/dL
CO₂ = 26 mEq/L	WBC = 6.3 × 10³/mm³	AST = 18 U/L
BUN = 12 mg/dL		ALT = 22 U/L
SCr = 1.3 mg/dL		T Bili = 0.2 mg/dL
Glu = 108 mg/dL		Alk Phos = 40 IU/L

Diagnostic Tests

▶ *Echocardiogram*

Ejection fraction 32%

QUESTIONS

1. Which of the following is the most common misconception about medication adherence?
   A. It is the provider's role to primarily manage a patient's chronic disease state
   B. Patients must have a sufficient understanding of the regimen
   C. Cultural factors may contribute to nonadherence
   D. Adherence can be assessed by both subjective and objective means

2. The term "adherence" refers to:
   A. The number of pills picked up from the pharmacy, and is economically focused
   B. The shared decision-making between the provider and the patient
   C. Passive behavior in which the patient is following instructions from the provider
   D. Active, voluntary, and collaborative involvement in a mutually accepted therapeutic course

3. What primary type of nonadherence is JW demonstrating?
   A. Capricious nonadherence
   B. Intelligent nonadherence
   C. Unintentional nonadherence
   D. Unintelligent nonadherence

4. Which of the following is a commonly known risk factor that may be contributing to his nonadherence?
   A. Hyperlipidemia diagnosis
   B. History of substance abuse
   C. Living alone
   D. Job instability

5. The following are behavioral interventions a provider could address and could benefit JW's medication adherence *EXCEPT*:
   A. Confirm administration technique
   B. Use adherence aids
   C. Increase the frequency of visits
   D. Simplify the treatment regimen
   E. Enlist the help of his partner

6. Which of the following requirements for medication adherence is JW missing for the carvedilol?
   A. Sufficient understanding of the disease and its associated medications
   B. Self-motivation to take the medication
   C. Implementation of necessary behavior changes
   D. None of the above

7. What side effect of furosemide is likely causing JW's nonadherence to this medication?
   A. Dry mouth
   B. Hypokalemia
   C. Constipation
   D. Diuresis

8. What is an appropriate alternative for carvedilol which would decrease JW's pill burden?
   A. Losartan 50 mg daily
   B. Metoprolol succinate 100 mg daily
   C. Propranolol 20 mg bid
   D. Amlodipine 10 mg daily

9. Which of the following would be a good adherence tool for a provider to recommend for JW?
   A. Cell phone medication application
   B. Weekly pill box
   C. Bedside alarm clock
   D. Pill bottle with dose counter lid

REFERENCES

1. Herrier RN, Apgar DA, Boyce RW, et al. Dealing with patient adherence issues. In: *Patient Assessment in Pharmacy*. New York, NY: McGraw-Hill; 2015. Accessed May 27, 2020.

2. Ho PM, Bryson CL, Rumsfeld JS. Medication adherence: its importance in cardiovascular outcomes. *Circulation*. 2009;119(23):3028-3035.

10 Cultural Considerations during Care Transitions

Elizabeth Haftel   Phung C. On

BACKGROUND

In healthcare, we often encounter patients from various cultural and religious backgrounds. It is important for pharmacists to understand how cultural and religious beliefs influence how patients manage their health. For many patients, religion, culture, and ethnicity play a major role in the decisions they make about their health.[1] People of some cultural and religious backgrounds may not understand the importance of taking potentially life-saving Western medications, going to see their doctor, or value the advice of others. Furthermore, patients with different belief systems may have varying opinions of the efficacy of Western medications and medical practices. By respecting the culture of our patients and asking them about their beliefs, healthcare providers can build a bond with patients and gain their trust.[1]

Many patients who are of Chinese descent focus on the concept of yin and yang, a balance of physical health and mind, also called qi or chi.[2] They believe that their mental health is most important and determines their overall physical health.[2] If patient believes that a medication is not working or causes a side effect, they will reduce the dose on their own or discontinue a medication rather than offend their doctor and voice their opinion.[2]

In this case, the pharmacist encounters a patient who practices traditional Chinese medicine and has medication adherence issues.

PATIENT PRESENTATION

Chief Complaint

My PCP retired, and I saw my new PCP 2 weeks ago to establish care. She said I might need some extra help with my medications.

History of Present Illness

FP is a 66-year-old female patient of Chinese descent. She immigrated to the United States 6 years ago with her husband to live with her daughter, son-in-law, and three grandchildren. Although she speaks some broken English, FP greatly relies on her daughter and son-in-law as translators at all of her appointments. She has an upcoming home visit scheduled with the clinic pharmacist following a transfer to a new primary care provider. FP's previous PCP stated that he has a hard time controlling FP's blood pressure because of medication adherence issues, mostly because of her profound beliefs in Chinese herbal medicines. He also states that FP has had multiple issues with her stomach, and this is a point of contention with this patient.

Past Medical History

Hypertension
GERD
Osteoarthritis
Peptic ulcer disease

Surgical History

Unknown; patient's daughter does not think that she had any surgical procedures

Family History

Mother: died at age 82 of "bad heart"
Father: died at age 77 of "bad brain"

Social History

Originally from China. Immigrated to US 6 years ago with husband.
Married with four adult children.
Lives with daughter, her husband, and three grandchildren.

Immunization

Up to date

Insurance

Medicare with additional Part C and D coverage

Patient does not report any difficulty affording her medications at this time

Allergies

No known drug allergies

Medication List from 1 year ago

- Lisinopril 20 mg, 1 tablet PO daily
- Ranitidine 150 mg, 1 tablet PO twice daily
- Omeprazole 40 mg, 1 capsule PO daily
- Alendronate 70 mg, 1 tablet PO every week

Current Medication List from PCP appointment 2 weeks ago

- Lisinopril 20 mg, 1 tablet PO daily
- Amlodipine 5 mg, 1 tablet PO daily
- Ranitidine 150 mg, 1 tablet PO twice daily
- Pantoprazole 40 mg, 1 tablet PO daily
- Sucralfate suspension 1 g, 1 tablet PO four times a day
- Alendronate 70 mg, 1 tablet PO every week

Physical Examination

▶ Vital Signs

Temp 98.2°F, HR 78, RR 23, BP 148/88 mmHg, Ht: 5′, Wt: 51 kg

▶ General

Well appearing older female in no acute distress.
All other systems are normal. Patient has new acute complaints.

Laboratory Findings from 2 weeks ago

Na = 138 mEq/L	Glu = 81 mg/dL
Cl = 98 mmol/dL	Mg = 1.8 mg/dL
K = 3.7 mEq/L	Ca = 8.2 mg/dL
BUN = 14 mg/dL	HbA1c = 5.3%
HCO = 25 mmol/L	

QUESTIONS

1. When you are completing a medication reconciliation using the medication lists above, what are some concerns regarding FP's medication list?
   A. Drug–drug interaction between lisinopril and alendronate
   B. Drug–drug interaction between ranitidine and pantoprazole
   C. No indication for alendronate in the patient's past medical history
   D. Patient is not taking any medications for the treatment of GERD

2. You arrive at FP's home to go over her medication regimen and you ask her family members to participate in the discussion. FP's daughter reports that her mother frequently requests refills on her alendronate, but they are often too early to refill the prescription through the insurance at the pharmacy. FP's daughter does not understand what the issue is since her mother is taking this medication daily as instructed by her previous PCP. What concerns do you have regarding FP's attempt at refilling her alendronate too soon?
   A. FP cannot afford to pay the out-of-pocket/cash price of alendronate
   B. FP is not taking her medication at all, putting her at higher risk of fractures
   C. FP is taking alendronate more frequently than prescribed, putting her at an increased risk of adverse drug events
   D. FP suspects that her stomach issue is getting worse, and decides to increase her dose of alendronate to protect her stomach

3. On discussion with FP and her family, it is found that FP does not like taking her prescribed medications because she prefers traditional Chinese medicine to resolve her ailments. She does not take all of her prescribed medications daily and relies on acupuncture and herbal medicine.
   When examining her medication cabinet, you see that the FP has multiple full bottles of lisinopril, dating back to 2 years ago. She states that it makes her cough, but she was afraid to tell anyone about the cough because she didn't want to offend her doctor. Studies have shown that elderly Chinese patients are less likely to report experiencing side effects, and self-discontinue medications rather than express concerns to providers.[2,3]
   Based on this conversation, what is the most likely cause for FP's blood pressure being uncontrolled at her last doctor's appointment?
   A. FP is not refilling the lisinopril prescription consistently due to cost issues.
   B. FP is not taking the lisinopril due to side effects. This is evident from the multiple full bottles present in the patient's home.
   C. FP is taking too much of her medication, resulting in inconsistent blood pressure control.
   D. FP lost her prescription insurance and cannot pick up her medications.

4. FP's new PCP added amlodipine to her antihypertensive regimen at the last office visit. He also told FP to continue taking lisinopril. If FP resumes lisinopril and starts amlodipine, why could this plan lead to an adverse drug event?
   A. FP is at risk of hypotension if she takes lisinopril and amlodipine together
   B. FP is at risk of hyperkalemia if she takes lisinopril and amlodipine together
   C. FP is at risk of rebound hypertension if she takes lisinopril and amlodipine together
   D. FP is not expected to experience any ADE if she takes lisinopril and amlodipine together

5. FP's blood pressure was taken multiple times throughout the home visit. At the beginning of the home visit, her blood pressure was 148/88 mmHg. Twenty minutes later, her blood pressure was 135/82 mmHg. Which of the following intervention(s) would be appropriate to manage FP's hypertension?

A. Discontinue all antihypertensive medication as the patient does not have hypertension

B. Discontinue lisinopril as the patient experienced unwanted side effects from the medication

C. Place the patient on a strict low sodium diet

D. Add metoprolol 25 mg, 1 tablet PO daily

6. FP is concerned that if she continues to take amlodipine, it can cause more problems, similar to lisinopril. FP states that even though she has not had any problems with amlodipine yet, she does not want to continue taking it. She would rather take Chinese herbal medicine since it is more natural. Which of the following motivational interviewing statements is MOST APPROPRIATE for FP in regard to her statement about taking herbal medicine instead of amlodipine?

A. "It is important for you to take this medication to lower your blood pressure or you will die from a heart attack."

B. "You can stop taking amlodipine if you are taking herbal medicine instead."

C. "You may not experience any side effects from amlodipine since you are tolerating it well right now. It is important to continue taking this medication to lower your blood pressure to prevent a heart attack or stroke."

D. "Amlodipine is cheaper than herbal medicine, so if you take amlodipine, it will save you money in the long run."

7. FP keeps a lot of Chinese herbal medicine in her medicine cabinet. She keeps a large amount of da suan and reports taking it 3 times a day. After researching da suan and recognizing that it is related to garlic, you find that it can potentially cause GI upset and irritation of the gut mucosa.[4] How could this potentially affect KP's health?

A. Drug–drug interactions could occur between herbal medicines and patients' prescribed medications

B. Herbal medicines are expensive

C. Herbal medicines are okay for this patient to take because they are natural products and cannot affect prescription medications

D. The patient should avoid all herbal medicines as they are all bad

REFERENCES

1. AHRQ. Health Literacy Precautions Toolkit, 2nd ed. Consider Culture, Customs, and Beliefs: Tool #10. Available at https://www.ahrq.gov/health-literacy/quality-resources/tools/literacy-toolkit/healthlittoolkit2-tool10.html. February 2015. Retrieved July 24, 2020.

2. Jin L, Acharya L. Cultural beliefs underlying medication adherence in people of Chinese descent in the United States. *Health Commun.* 2015;31(5):513-521.

3. Hsu Y-H, Mao C-L, Wey M. Antihypertensive medication adherence among elderly Chinese Americans. *J Transcult Nurs.* 2010;21(4):297-305.

4. Blumenthal M, Busse WE, Goldberg A, et al. eds. *The Complete German Commission E Monographs: Therapeutic Guide to Herbal Medicines.* Boston: Integrative Medicine Communications; 1998.

Section 3

Patients with Diabetes

11 Hyperglycemic Crisis: Diabetic Ketoacidosis in Type 1 Diabetes

Kimberly Won   Jelena Lewis
Laressa Bethishou

PATIENT PRESENTATION

Chief Complaint

"I feel weak and am short of breath."

History of Present Illness

PJ is a 23-year-old Caucasian female who is brought to the emergency department (ED) by her mother for generalized weakness and deep, labored breathing. She complains of having polyuria, polydipsia, diminished appetite, nausea and vomiting, and abdominal pain for the past 2 to 3 days. Patient denies fever, chills, heartburn, melena, hematemesis, diarrhea, or constipation.

Patient states that she was diagnosed with diabetes mellitus type 1 about 3 months ago, at which time she received prescriptions for insulin degludec, insulin lispro, and lisinopril. She admits to not picking up the insulin degludec due to cost. However, she does have insulin lispro and lisinopril at home. She states that she has been taking her lisinopril, but not her insulin lispro. At this previous visit, she was also instructed to schedule an appointment with an endocrinologist and a registered dietitian; however, she has not done either.

Past Medical History

Type 1 diabetes mellitus, microalbuminuria

Surgical History

None

Family History

Father with type 1 diabetes

Social History

Lives with her parents

Occasional EtOH use (drinks socially on the weekends). Denies tobacco use.

Immunization

Up-to-date with childhood vaccinations, including hepatitis B vaccination series

Insurance

Aetna HMO

Allergies

No known drug allergies

Home Medications

- Insulin degludec 15 units subcutaneous every day at bedtime
- Insulin lispro 5 units subcutaneous every day prior to each meal
- Lisinopril 10 mg PO daily
- Nexplanon® 65 mg subdermal (inserted 6 months ago)

Physical Examination

▶ *Vital Signs*

Temp 98.1°F, HR 118 bpm, RR 28 breaths per min, BP 88/64 mmHg, O_2 sat 92%, Ht: 5'5", Wt: 54.5 kg

▶ *General*

Altered, lethargic female

▶ *HEENT*

Normocephalic, PERRLA, EOMI

► *Pulmonary*

SOB, (+) Kussmaul respirations, fruity breath

► *Cardiovascular*

Tachycardic, hypotensive, weak pulse, NSR, no m/r/g

► *Abdomen*

Mild abdominal tenderness, (+) bowel sounds

► *Neurologic*

Drowsy and altered, A&O × 2 (person and place)

► *Extremities*

Dry mucous membranes, poor skin turgor, increased capillary refill time

Laboratory Findings

Chemistry	Arterial Blood Gas	Urine Analysis
Na^+ 133 mEq/L	pH 7.15	Urine cloudy
K^+ 4.8 mEq/L	pO_2 45 mmHg	pH 5.5
Cl^- 96 mEq/L	pCO_2 25 mmHg	Specific gravity
CO_2 9 mEq/L	HCO_3 8 mEq/L	1.031
BUN 45 mg/dL		(+) Ketones
SCr 1.4 mg/dL		(−) Nitrates
Glucose 397 mg/dL		(−) Leukocyte
Mg^{2+} 2.0 mg/dL		esterase
Ca^{2+} 9.4 mg/dL		(+) Protein
Phos 4.3 mg/dL		(+) Glucose
Total cholesterol:		
214 mg/dL		
LDL: 131 mg/dL		
HDL: 36 mg/dL		
Triglycerides:		
235 mg/dL		
Hemoglobin A1c:		
12.3%		
From previous encounter Albumin/Cr: 220 mg/g		

Diagnostic Tests

► *Chest X-Ray*

Normal

► *Electrocardiogram*

Sinus tachycardia

Emergency Department Course

23-year-old female presented to the ED with diabetic ketoacidosis (DKA). In the ED, she was given 1.5 L Lactated Ringers IV bolus (at 999 mL/h), followed by an IV infusion of a liter of half-normal saline (at 200 mL/h) and potassium chloride 20 mEq IV. Patient was started on regular insulin per the hospital's DKA protocol. She received 5.5 units insulin regular IV bolus, followed by a continuous IV infusion of insulin regular (at 5.5 units/h). After 4 hours, the patient was transferred to the intensive care unit (ICU) for further care. At that time, her point-of-care glucose was 266 mg/dL and repeat vitals were: Temp 98.4°F, HR 92 bpm, RR 21 breaths per min, BP 109/78 mmHg.

QUESTIONS

1. After transferring to the ICU, the patient's repeat labs are Na^+ 134 mEq/L, K^+ 4.6 mEq/L, Cl^- 100 mEq/L, CO_2 13 mEq/L, BUN 35 mg/dL, SCr 1.5 mg/dL, glucose 242 mg/dL. Which medications would be most appropriate to order for PJ while she is admitted to the ICU?
   A. 0.9% NaCl infusion, insulin regular IV infusion per DKA protocol, lisinopril 10 mg PO daily, sodium bicarbonate 100 mEq IV, potassium 20 mEq IV, enoxaparin 30 mg subcutaneous daily
   B. 0.45% NaCl infusion, subcutaneous insulin aspart per DKA protocol, enoxaparin 30 mg subcutaneous daily, pantoprazole 40 mg IV daily
   C. 0.45% NaCl/D5W infusion, insulin regular infusion per DKA protocol, enoxaparin 40 mg subcutaneous daily, potassium 20 mEq IV
   D. 0.45% NaCl/D5W infusion, insulin aspart subcutaneous per DKA protocol, lisinopril 10 mg PO daily, enoxaparin 40 mg subcutaneous daily, potassium 20 mEq IV

2. After PJ's DKA has resolved and she is eating a full diet, the ICU team would like to transition PJ from IV insulin to a subcutaneous insulin formulation on formulary. Using weight-based dosing, what would be the most appropriate subcutaneous regimen to transition PJ to?
   A. Insulin glargine 24 units subcutaneous once daily and insulin aspart 4 units subcutaneous with meals
   B. Insulin degludec 15 units subcutaneous once daily and insulin lispro 5 units subcutaneous with meals
   C. Insulin glargine 21 units subcutaneous once daily and insulin aspart 7 units subcutaneous with meals
   D. Insulin degludec 30 units subcutaneous once daily and insulin lispro 10 units subcutaneous with meals

3. Instead of using weight-based insulin dosing, the physician would like to start a subcutaneous insulin regimen based on PJ's insulin drip rate (listed below). Which would be the most appropriate subcutaneous insulin regimen to transition PJ to?

Time	1900	2000	2100	2200	2300	0000	0100	0200	0300	0400	0500	0600	0700	0800	0900
BG (mg/dL)	230	204	196	176	168	156	150	143	148	150	141	144	152	143	147
Insulin infusion (units/ hr)	4	3	3	2	3	2	3	2	2	3	2	2	3	2	2

    A. Insulin glargine 24 units subcutaneous once daily plus insulin lispro 8 units subcutaneous with meals

    B. Insulin glargine 14 units subcutaneous once daily plus high-intensity sliding scale insulin with meals

    C. Insulin glargine 28 units subcutaneous once daily plus insulin lispro 9 units subcutaneous with meals

    D. Insulin glargine 10 units subcutaneous at bedtime plus a high-intensity sliding scale insulin with meals

4. Which is the most appropriate timing strategy to transition from the continuous insulin infusion to subcutaneous insulin?

    A. Stop the insulin infusion and then immediately administer the long-acting insulin subcutaneous

    B. Stop the insulin infusion and administer the long-acting insulin subcutaneous 2 hours after the end of the infusion

    C. Administer the long-acting insulin subcutaneous and stop the insulin infusion 2 hours after

    D. Administer the long-acting insulin subcutaneous and then immediately stop the insulin infusion

5. Once the patient's DKA and acute kidney injury are resolved, the patient is transferred to the medicine floor. Prior to discharge, the patient and her parents are provided with education on type 1 diabetes and the importance of injecting insulin every day. The patient receives several consults with a registered dietitian who extensively discussed how to use a glucometer and record self-monitoring blood glucose reading, when to check sugars, and how to incorporate dietary modifications to help lower her A1c.

    Based on the ADA 2020 guidelines, what outpatient glycemic targets for preprandial and 1- to 2-hour postprandial (PPD) blood glucose (BG) should be set with PJ prior to discharge?

    A. Preprandial BG: <110 mg/dL, 1-2 hour PPD BG: <140 mg/dL

    B. Preprandial BG: 80−130 mg/dL, 1-2 hour PPD BG: <180 mg/dL

    C. Preprandial BG: 70−130 mg/dL, 1-2 hour PPD BG: 110−140 mg/dL

    D. Preprandial BG: 80−130 mg/dL, 1-2 hour PPD BG: <140 mg/dL

6. Provided that PJ is up-to-date with all of her childhood vaccines in addition to the influenza vaccine, which other vaccines would you recommend for PJ prior to discharge?

    A. Hepatitis B vaccine

    B. Pneumococcal conjugate vaccine (PCV13)

    C. Shingles vaccine

    D. Pneumococcal polysaccharide vaccine (PPSV23)

7. Which medication regimen should the patient be discharged with?

    A. Lisinopril 10 mg daily, insulin degludec 15 units subcutaneous every day at bedtime, insulin lispro 5 units subcutaneous every day prior to each meal, atorvastatin 20 mg daily, pantoprazole 40 mg daily

    B. Lisinopril 10 mg daily, insulin glargine 24 units subcutaneous every day at bedtime, insulin lispro 8 units subcutaneous every day prior to each meal

    C. Insulin glargine 24 units subcutaneous every day at bedtime, insulin lispro 8 units subcutaneous every day prior to each meal, atorvastatin 20 mg daily, pantoprazole 40 mg daily

    D. Lisinopril 10 mg daily, insulin glargine 28 units subcutaneous every day at bedtime, insulin lispro 5 units subcutaneous every day prior to each meal, atorvastatin 20 mg daily

8. Once PJ is discharged, which healthcare providers should PJ follow up with and when should this follow-up occur?

    A. Nephrologist, endocrinologist, and primary care provider in 1 to 2 weeks

    B. Primary care provider, endocrinologist, and diabetes educator in 1 to 2 weeks

    C. Primary care provider, endocrinologist, and diabetes educator in 1 month

    D. Nephrologist, endocrinologist, and diabetes educator in 1 month

9. In addition to carbohydrate counting, blood glucose meter and insulin injection teaching, what are other important education points for this patient when providing discharge counseling?

    A. Hypoglycemia management

    B. Adherence to medications

    C. Lisinopril discontinuation during pregnancy

    D. All of the above

REFERENCES

1. Kitabachi AE, Umpierrez GE, Miles JM, et al. Hyperglycemic crises in adult patients with diabetes. *Diabetes Care*. 2009;32(7):1335-1343.

2. American Diabetes Association. Hyperglycemic crises in diabetes. *Diabetes Care*. 2004;27(suppl 1):s94-s102.

3. Umpierrez G, Korytkowski M. Diabetic emergencies – ketoacidosis, hyperglycaemic hyperosmolar state and hypoglycaemia. *Nat Rev Endocrinol*. 2016;12(4):222-232.

4. American Diabetes Association. Diabetes Care in the Hospital: Standards of Medical Care in Diabetes — 2021. *Diabetes Care*. 2021;44(suppl 1):S211-S220.

5. Hillier TA, Abbott RD, Barrett EJ. Hyponatremia: evaluating the correction factor for hyperglycemia. *Am J Med*. 1999;106(4):399-403.

6. Katz MA. Hyperglycemia-induced hyponatremia – calculation of expected serum sodium depression. *N Engl J Med*. 1973;289(16):843-844.

7. Gerotziafas GT, Papageorgiou L, Salta S, et al. Updated clinical models for VTE prediction in hospitalized medical patients. *Thromb Res*. 2018;164(suppl 1):S62-S69.

8. Kahn SR, Lim W, Dunn AS, et al. Prevention of VTE in non-surgical patients. *Chest*. 2012;141(2 suppl):e195S-e226S.

9. Cook D, Guyatt G. Prophylaxis against upper gastrointestinal bleeding in hospitalized patients. *N Engl J Med*. 2018;378:2506-2516.

10. Moghissi ES, Korytkowski MT, DiNardo M, et al. American Association of Clinical Endocrinologists and American Diabetes Association consensus statement on inpatient glycemic control. *Diabetes Care*. 2009;32(6):1119-1131.

11. Avanzini F, Marelli G, Donzelli W, et al. Transition from intravenous to subcutaneous insulin. *Diabetes Care*. 2011;34(7):1445-1450.

12. Degludec [package insert]. Plainsboro, NJ: Novo Nordisk Inc. 2015.

13. Lantus [package insert]. Bridgewater, NJ: Sanofi-Aventis. 2009.

14. American Diabetes Association. Glycemic targets: standards of medical care in diabetes — 2021. *Diabetes Care*. 2021;44(suppl 1):S111-S124.

15. The NICE-SUGAR Investigators. Intensive versus conventional glucose control in critically ill patients. *N Engl J Med*. 2009;360:1283-1297.

16. Handelsman Y, Bloomgarden ZT, Grunberger G, et al. American Association of Clinical Endocrinologists and American College of Endocrinology — clinical practice guidelines for developing a diabetes mellitus comprehensive care plan — 2015. *Endocr Pract*. 2015;(suppl 1):1-87.

17. American Diabetes Association. Comprehensive medical evaluation and assessment of comorbidities: standards of medical care in diabetes — 2021. *Diabetes Care*. 2021;44(suppl 1):S40-S52.

18. Centers for Disease Control and Prevention. Vaccines and Preventable Diseases. https://www.cdc.gov/vaccines/vpd/index.html. Bethesda, MD. 2020.

19. American Diabetes Association. Cardiovascular disease and risk management: standards for medical care in diabetes – 2021. *Diabetes Care*. 2021;44(suppl 1):S125-S150.

20. American Diabetes Association. Management of diabetes in pregnancy: standards for medical care in diabetes – 2021. *Diabetes Care*. 2021;44(suppl 1):S200-S210.

Microvascular Complications of Diabetes: Peripheral Neuropathy

Nikhil A. Sangave   Phung C. On

PATIENT PRESENTATION

Chief Complaint

"I've been waking up at night with a burning and tingling feeling in my fingers and toes."

History of Present Illness

AP is a 64-year-old African American male who presents to the primary care clinic with a glucometer and medication list. The patient states that he has been adherent to his medications including insulin glargine, metformin, and his newly prescribed dulaglutide. The patient states that he has been attempting to "live healthier" by jogging 30 minutes at least four times a week and minimizing fast food. Of note, the patient reports experiencing distal symmetric peripheral neuropathy (DSPN) over the last year in the tips of his fingers and toes that wakes him up at night. The patient also states that he has been experiencing bloating, nausea, and vomiting over the past 6 months, however the vomiting has become more pronounced over the past 3 months, especially after eating meals.

Past Medical History

Type 2 diabetes (diagnosed 2001)
Hypertension
Dyslipidemia
s/p STEMI (2015)

Surgical History

CABG (2015)

Family History

Mother: history of T2DM, alive at 96 years of age
Father: HTN, deceased
No siblings
No children

Social History

Lives with wife of 30 years.
Drinks beer occasionally.
No cigarette or recreational drug use.

Immunization

Up to date

Insurance

Medicaid

Allergies

Aspirin (anaphylaxis)

Home Medications

- Atorvastatin 40 mg, 1 tablet PO daily
- Clopidogrel 75 mg, 1 tablet PO daily
- Insulin glargine 100 units/mL, 32 units SC QPM
- Dulaglutide 0.75 mg/0.5 mL, 0.75 mg SC once weekly (initiated 2 months ago)
- Amlodipine 5 mg, 1 tablet PO daily
- Levothyroxine 50 mcg, 1 tablet PO daily
- Losartan 100 mg, 1 tablet PO daily
- Metformin 1000 mg, 1 tablet PO bid
- Metoprolol succinate, 1 tablet 50 mg daily
- Multivitamin, 1 tablet PO daily

Physical Examination

▶ *Vital Signs*

Temp 99.1, P 78, RR 18, BP 128/86 mmHg, Ht: 5′9″, Wt: 185 lbs

▶ *General*

Well-nourished male.

► **HEENT**

PERRLA, EOMI.
No sore throat, oral ulcers or pain, or trouble swallowing.
No change in hearing/vision.

► **Pulmonary**

CTAB. No cough or shortness of breath.

► **Cardiovascular**

RRR, no m/r/g.

► **Abdomen**

Soft, +BS, some tenderness.

► **Genitourinary**

Deferred.

► **Neurologic**

Deferred.

► **Extremities**

No edema, 2+ distal pulses.

Laboratory Findings (drawn 2 weeks ago)

Na = 135 mEq/L	Hgb = 14.4 g/dL	Ca = 9.0 mg/dL
K = 3.9 mEq/L	Hct = 43%	Mg = 2.3 mEq/L
Cl = 102 mEq/L	Plt = 137×10^3 /μL	Phos = 3.3 mg/dL
CO_2 = 22 mEq/L	WBC = 4.2×10^3 /μL	AST = 16 IU/L
BUN = 14 mg/dL		ALT = 19 IU/L
SCr = 0.9 mg/dL		T Bili = 0.1 mg/dL
Glu = 142 mg/dL		Alk Phos = 75 IU/L

Most recent thyroid panel

Total T4	8.3 mcg/dL
T3	94 ng/dL
TSH	3.1 microunits/mL

Most recent lipid panel

Total cholesterol	146 mg/dL
Triglycerides	86 mg/dL
HDL	51 mg/dL
LDL	78 mg/dL

Most recent A1c: 7.6%
Most recent vitamin B_{12} level: 300 ng/mL
Self-monitored blood glucose averages (past 1 month):

Fasting Blood Glucose (n = 27)	Before Lunch (n = 12)	2 h After Dinner/ Bedtime (n = 14)
141 mg/dL	162 mg/dL	200 mg/dL

QUESTIONS

1. During triage, the nurse interviews AP to obtain a medication history. AP reports taking all of his medications every day in the morning with breakfast except for the medications he has to inject. He injects his insulin glargine in the evening every day and his dulaglutide every Monday. After completing a medication reconciliation using the medication history obtained from the triage nurse and the prescribed medication list in the EHR, you were able to identify which of the following medication-related problem(s)?
   A. AP is taking atorvastatin incorrectly
   B. AP is taking levothyroxine incorrectly
   C. AP is taking dulaglutide incorrectly
   D. All of the above

2. Which of the following is NOT in the differential diagnosis for *diabetic* peripheral neuropathy?
   A. Thyroid disorder
   B. Vitamin B_{12} deficiency
   C. Vitamin K deficiency
   D. Chronic amiodarone use

3. Which of the following is NOT a potential sign or symptom associated with cardiovascular autonomic neuropathy (CAN)?
   A. Syncope
   B. Anhidrosis
   C. Resting tachycardia
   D. Orthostatic hypotension

4. What are appropriate counseling points for gabapentin when used for peripheral neuropathy?
   A. Do not abruptly discontinue this medication as serious effects may occur
   B. Do not drive or operate heavy machinery until the full effects of the medication are realized
   C. Report any signs of worsening mood or suicidal ideation
   D. All of the above

5. What may be the most likely causes of AP's frequent vomiting, bloating, and nausea?
   A. Gastroparesis and dulaglutide
   B. Gastroparesis and metformin
   C. Esophageal dysfunction and metformin
   D. Esophageal dysfunction and dulaglutide

6. Which medication regimen would be most appropriate for AP's neuropathy at this time?
   A. Tapentadol ER 50 mg PO bid
   B. Amitriptyline 25 mg PO daily
   C. Pregabalin 25 mg PO daily
   D. Venlafaxine 37.5 mg PO daily

7. Which of the following is true regarding the use of duloxetine for DSPN?
   A. Duloxetine is not FDA approved for any type of diabetic neuropathy
   B. Duloxetine may lead to insomnia, anorexia, and/or sexual side effects
   C. Duloxetine may suppress breathing
   D. Duloxetine should be taken three times daily

8. AP arrives at his local retail pharmacy to pick up his medications, including his new prescription for pregabalin for peripheral neuropathy. He realizes that the copay for the medication is far more than he can afford. He calls your clinic and asks for advice. What is a more cost-effective medication for AP's peripheral neuropathy?
   A. Tapentadol ER 50 mg PO bid
   B. Nortriptyline 25 mg PO daily
   C. Gabapentin 100 mg PO tid
   D. Tramadol 50 mg bid

9. Which of AP's medications should be modified due to peripheral neuropathy?
   A. Insulin glargine
   B. Metformin
   C. Dulaglutide
   D. Metoprolol succinate

10. AP's PCP decides to discontinue his dulaglutide and after 3 months and his A1c rises to 7.9% despite following a rigid diet and exercise routine. AP's PCP decides to refer him to endocrinology to manage his diabetes. What medication would be most appropriate at this time to help AP reduce his A1c?
    A. Insulin aspart
    B. Dapagliflozin
    C. Semaglutide
    D. Pioglitazone

REFERENCES

1. American Diabetes Association. Microvascular complications and foot care: standards of medical care in diabetes – 2020. *Diabetes Care.* 2020;43(suppl 1):S135-S151.
2. Pop-Busui R, Boulton A, Feldman EL, et al. Diabetic Neuropathy: A Position Statement by the American Diabetes Association. *American Diabetes Association.* 2017;40:136-154.

13 Macrovascular Complications of Diabetes: Acute Kidney Injury

Rebecca L. Dunn   Jessica Wooster
Winter J. Smith

PATIENT PRESENTATION

Chief Complaint

"I think I have the flu."

History of Present Illness

KJ is a 76-year-old African American female who presents to the ED from a senior living community with complaints of vomiting, diarrhea, and feeling unwell. She states that she became ill 4 days prior to admission, and has been vomiting every few hours, having watery diarrhea five times per day, and has body aches and subjective fever. The provider at the senior living community visited her 3 days prior to arrival and instructed her to drink plenty of fluids and take over-the-counter analgesics for aches and pains. However, she states that she has had a poor appetite and has not felt well enough to eat or drink. Other than her maintenance medications, she has been taking two over-the-counter ibuprofen tablets every 4 to 6 hours since her visit with the facility's provider. She also reports decreased urination, but thinks it is probably due to her poor oral intake.

Past Medical History

T2 DM
CKD [baseline SCr 1.1 (3 days prior)]
HTN [baseline BP 124/76 mmHg (3 days prior)]
GERD

Family History

Mother: T2DM, HLD, HTN, obesity, and died at age 81 from an ischemic stroke
Father: HTN, died in MVA at age 68
Sibling: T2DM, HTN (living)

Social History

Negative for tobacco, alcohol, and illicit drug use.

Immunization

Up to date

Insurance

Aetna PPO

Allergies

No known drug allergies

Home Medications

- Metformin 1000 mg PO bid
- Glipizide IR 10 mg PO daily
- Lisinopril/HCTZ 20 mg/12.5 mg, 2 tablets PO daily
- Metoprolol succinate 25 mg PO daily
- Famotidine 20 mg PO twice daily
- ASA 81 mg PO daily
- Ibuprofen 400 mg PO every 4–6 hours as needed for pain or fever

Physical Examination

▶ **Vital Signs**

Temp 99.7°F, P 120, RR 18, BP 88/56 mmHg, pO_2 94 %
Ht: 5′9″, Wt: 72 kg

▶ **General**

Appears stated age, in mild distress, pale and diaphoretic.

▶ **HEENT**

Normocephalic, atraumatic, PERRLA, EOMI, dry mucus membranes and conjunctiva, no neck stiffness/pain, no photophobia.

Conflict of Interest Disclosure: The author has no financial or other interest that may bias the production of this manuscript.

▸ *Pulmonary*

CTAB.

▸ *Cardiovascular*

Tachycardic, no m/r/g.

▸ *Abdomen*

Soft, non-distended, nontender to palpation, bowel sounds hyperactive.

▸ *Genitourinary*

Normal female genitalia, no complaints of dysuria or hematuria.

▸ *Neurologic*

A&O × 3, cranial nerves intact.

▸ *Extremities*

Normal range of motion, no edema, poor skin turgor, slow capillary refill, 2+ pulses.

▸ *Review of Systems*

Positive for headache in addition to symptoms described in History of Present Illness.

Laboratory Values (from ED)

Na = 147 mEq/L	Hgb = 12.5 g/dL	AST = 38 IU/L
K = 4.2 mEq/L	Hct = 37%	ALT = 25 IU/L
Cl = 97 mEq/L	Plt = 157 × 10^3/mm³	Alk Phos = 100 IU/L
CO_2 = 25 mEq/L	WBC = 8.1 × 10^3/mm³	Albumin = 4.0 g/dL
BUN = 64 mg/dL	Neutros = 65%	T Bili = 1.7 mg/dL
SCr = 2.5 mg/dL	Bands = 1%	Mg = 2.0 mg/dL
eGFR = 21 mL/min/1.73 m²	Lymphs = 20%	Phos = 3.1 mg/dL
Glu = 90 mg/dL	Monos = 3%	Ca = 10.2 mg/dL
A1c = 10%		

Urinalysis

RBC: negative	WBC: absent	Crystals: absent
Casts: absent	Epithelial cells: absent	Protein: 30 mg/g
pH: 6.7	Specific gravity: 1.008	Urine Na: 15 mEq/L
Ucr: 90 mg/dL	Glucose = Absent	Nitrite: positive
Color: yellow	Clarity = clear	
Leukocyte esterase: negative		
Urine osmolarity: 622 mOsm/kg		

Influenza Test

Negative.

Blood Cultures

No growth to date.

Urine cultures

Pending.

KJ is admitted to the general medical ward of the hospital for inpatient treatment. Admission orders have been written to continue home medications as previously prescribed.

QUESTIONS

1. According to the KDIGO Clinical Practice Guidelines for Acute Kidney Injury, what parameter most clearly defines KJ as having acute kidney injury (AKI)?
   A. Creatine clearance <30 mL/min
   B. Serum creatinine 1.5 times baseline
   C. ≥0.3 mg/dL decrease in serum creatinine
   D. < 0.5 mL/kg/h urine output for the last 12 hours

2. What susceptibility factor most likely contributed to KJ's development of AKI?
   A. Female gender
   B. Dehydration
   C. Age
   D. Chronic kidney disease (CKD)

3. What medication is not likely to have contributed to the development of KJ's AKI?
   A. Ibuprofen
   B. Metformin
   C. Lisinopril
   D. Hydrochlorothiazide

4. What is the most likely causative mechanism of KJ's AKI?
   A. Prerenal
   B. Intrinsic
   C. Acute tubular necrosis
   D. Obstructive

5. Which adjustment to KJ's home medications should be made based on her current renal function?
   A. Change glipizide to glyburide 10 mg once daily
   B. Discontinue aspirin
   C. Discontinue metformin
   D. Change metoprolol succinate to metoprolol tartrate

6. Which is the most appropriate strategy for management of KJ's diabetes while she is hospitalized?
   A. Continue sulfonylurea therapy
   B. Continue sulfonylurea and initiate sliding scale insulin
   C. Discontinue sulfonylurea and initiate basal insulin
   D. Discontinue sulfonylurea and initiate an SGLT2 inhibitor

7. KJ's vomiting and diarrhea resolved, and she is eating and drinking again. The medical team is preparing for hospital discharge and her post-discharge follow-up appointment has been scheduled. Her labs and vitals have been stable for the past 48 hours. Her current blood pressure is 152/94 mmHg, SCr is 1.1 mg/dL, and blood glucose is 210 mg/dL. Which is the most appropriate adjustment to KJ's home medication regimen to be implemented at discharge?
   A. Decrease metformin dose to 500 mg daily
   B. Decrease glipizide dose to 5 mg daily
   C. Increase aspirin dose to 325 mg daily
   D. Resume home lisinopril/HCTZ dose
   E. Replace ibuprofen with naproxen

8. Which is the most appropriate pharmacist recommendation to KJ for management of mild aches and pains after discharge?
   A. Use over-the-counter acetaminophen
   B. Use over-the-counter topical diclofenac
   C. Contact your PCP for a celecoxib prescription
   D. Contact your PCP for a hydrocodone prescription

9. What parameter should be evaluated at KJ's post-discharge follow-up appointment to monitor for the continued resolution of AKI?
   A. Urine output (UOP)
   B. Serum creatinine (SCr)
   C. GFR estimated by the Four-Variable Modification of Diet in Renal Disease Study (MDRD4) equation
   D. Creatinine clearance estimated by Cockcroft-Gault equation

10. While filling KJ's discharge medications, the community pharmacist notices that KJ's GERD therapy was changed from famotidine to omeprazole. This change is inappropriate for which of the following reasons?
   A. KJ's symptoms are currently uncontrolled with H2RA therapy
   B. PPIs are less potent inhibitors of gastric acid secretion than H2RAs
   C. H2RA use has been associated with fractures and bone loss
   D. PPI use has been associated with Clostridioides difficile infection

REFERENCES

1. Kellum JA, Lameire N, Aspelin P, et al. KDIGO clinical practice guidelines for acute kidney injury. *Kidney Int Suppl*. 2012;2:1-138.
2. Prieto-Garcia L, Pericacho M, Sancho-Martinex SM, et al. Mechanism of triple whammy acute kidney injury. *Pharmacol Therap*. 2016;167:132-145.
3. Lexicomp Online, Lexi-Drugs Online, Hudson, Ohio: Wolters Kluwer Clinical Drug Information, Inc.; 2020. Accessed June 2, 2020.
4. National Kidney Foundation. KDOQI clinical practice guideline for diabetes and CKD: 2012 update. *Am J Kidney Dis*. 2012;60:850-886.
5. American Diabetes Association. 12. Older adults: standards of medical care in diabetes - 2020. *Diabetes Care*. 2020;43(suppl 1):S152-S162.
6. National Kidney Foundation. KDOQI clinical practice guidelines and clinical practice recommendations for diabetes and chronic kidney disease. *Am J Kidney Dis*. 2007;49(suppl 2):S1-S180.
7. American Diabetes Association. 15. Diabetes care in the hospital: standards of medical care in diabetes - 2020. *Diabetes Care*. 2020;43(suppl 1):S193-S202.
8. Whelton PK, Carey RM, Aronow WS, et al. 2017 ACC/AHA/AAPA/ABC/ACPM/AGS/APhA/ASH/ASPC/NMA/PCNA guideline for the prevention, detection, evaluation, and management of high blood pressure in adults: a report of the American College of Cardiology/American Heart Association task force on clinical practice guidelines. *J Am Coll Cardiol*. 2018;71:e127-E148.
9. American Diabetes Association. 6. Glycemic targets: standards of medical care in diabetes - 2020. *Diabetes Care*. 2020;43(suppl 1):S66-S76.
10. Pham PC, Khaing K, Sievers TM, et al. 2017 update on pain management in patients with chronic kidney disease. *Clin Kidney J*. 2017;10:688-697.
11. Koncicki HM, Unruh M, Schell JO. Pain management in CKD: a guide for nephrology providers. *Am J Kidney Dis*. 2017;69:451-460.
12. Dowling TC. Evaluation of kidney function. In: DiPiro JT, Talbert RL, Yee GC, Matzke GR, Wells BG, Posey L, eds. *Pharmacotherapy: A Pathophysiologic Approach*. 10th ed. New York, NY: McGraw-Hill. http://accesspharmacy.mhmedical.com/content.aspx?bookid=1861&sectionid=134127006. Accessed June 3, 2020.
13. The 2019 American Geriatrics Society Beers Criteria® Update Expert Panel. American Geriatrics Society 2019 updated AGS Beers Criteria® for potentially inappropriate medication use in older adults. *J Am Geriatr Soc*. 2019;67:674-694.
14. Maes ML, Fixen DR, Linnebur SA. Adverse effects of proton-pump inhibitor use in older adults: a review of the evidence. *Ther Adv Drug Saf*. 2017;8:273-297.
15. Eom CK, Park SM, Myung SK, Yun JM, Ahn JS. Use of acid-suppressive drugs and risk of fracture: a meta-analysis of observational studies. *Ann Fam Med*. 2011;9:257-267.

Section 4

Patients with Cardiovascular Conditions

14 Acute Coronary Syndromes: Non-ST Elevated Myocardial Infarction

Erika Felix-Getzik   Phung C. On

PATIENT PRESENTATION

Chief Complaint

"I have been having chest pain off and on since waking up this morning."

History of Present Illness

KT is a 62-year-old white male who presents to the emergency department with intermittent 9/10 chest pressure that radiates to his left jaw and shoulder, nausea, shortness of breath, and dizziness. His symptoms started upon waking about 6 hours ago. He reports four episodes of discomfort since this morning that suddenly come and go; the episodes last no longer than 10 to 20 minutes. The patient is given aspirin (chewed) 325 mg by mouth × 1 and is started on oxygen, nitroglycerin (NTG) 5 mcg/min gtt, and enoxaparin 100 mg subcutaneously twice daily. Stat labs and an EKG are ordered.

Past Medical History

Depression
Diabetes mellitus (DM) type 2
Dyslipidemia
Hypertension (HTN)
Hypothyroidism
Osteoarthritis (bilateral knees)

Surgical History

Rotator cuff repair

Family History

Father had a myocardial infarction (MI) at 54 years old

Social History

Married with three daughters.
Works as a computer consultant.
Lives a sedentary life.
Drinks 1 to 2 bourbons per night.
Quit smoking 10 years ago (30 pack/year history).

Immunization

Up to date

Insurance

Blue Cross/Blue Shield

Allergies

Penicillin (hives)

Home Medications/supplements

- Atorvastatin 20 mg PO daily
- Glucosamine 1500 mg/chondroitin 1200 mg PO daily
- HCTZ 25 mg PO daily
- Ibuprofen 400 mg PO every 6 hours as needed knee pain
- Levothyroxine 88 mcg PO daily
- Lisinopril 20 mg PO daily
- Metformin ER 1000 mg PO daily
- Multivitamin PO daily
- Sertraline 50 mg PO daily
- Turmeric 100 mg PO daily

Physical Examination

▶ *Vital Signs*

Temp 97.6°F, P 116, RR 28, BP 162/102 mmHg, pO_2 98%, Ht: 6′1″, Wt: 100.4 kg

▶ *General*

Well nourished, overweight male in moderate distress.

▸ *HEENT*

PERRLA, EOMI.

▸ *Pulmonary*

Increased respirations, lungs are clear to auscultation bilaterally.

▸ *Cardiovascular*

Tachycardic, t-wave inversions in lateral leads, no m/r/g.

▸ *Abdomen*

Soft, non-distended, nontender, normal bowel sounds.

▸ *Genitourinary*

Normal male genitalia, no complaints of dysuria or hematuria.

▸ *Neurologic*

Alert and oriented to person, place, and time.

▸ *Extremities*

No edema, peripheral pulses intact.

Laboratory Findings

Na = 140 mEq/L	Plt = 135 × 10^3/mm^3	ALT = 38 IU/L
K = 4.2 mEq/L	WBC = 6 × 10^3/mm^3	T Bili = 1.6 mg/dL
Cl = 101 mEq/L	cTnT = 0.6 ng/mL	Alk Phos = 160 IU/L
CO_2 = 27 mEq/L	CK = 325 U/L	Total Chol = 202 mg/dL
BUN = 22 mg/dL	CK-MB = 38 U/L	LDL-C = 102 mg/dL
SCr = 1.02 mg/dL	BNP = 74 pg/mL	HDL-C = 42 mg/dL
Glu = 132 mg/dL	Ca = 8.9 mg/dL	Trig = 187 mg/dL
Hgb = 14.9 g/dL	Mg = 1.8 mg/dL	HgbA1c = 6.7%
Hct = 40%	AST = 46 IU/L	TSH = 1.43 mIU/L

Diagnostic Tests

▸ *Electrocardiogram*

HR 108 bpm, t-wave inversions in anterior leads

▸ *Echocardiogram*

EF = 62%, no wall motion abnormalities

▸ *Cardiac Catheterization*

90% occlusion of the left anterior descending artery (LAD); angioplasty performed, and drug-eluting stent (DES) placed

QUESTIONS

1. What laboratory test(s) help identify a patient with MI?
   A. Elevated cTnT T (>0.4 ng/mL)
   B. Elevated CK (>200 U/L)
   C. Elevated CK-MB (>25 U/L)
   D. All of the above

2. Based on KT's presentation, risk factors, EKG, and cardiac biomarkers, what is his probable diagnosis?
   A. Stable angina
   B. Unstable angina
   C. Non-ST-elevation myocardial infarction (NSTEMI)
   D. ST-elevation myocardial infarction (STEMI)

3. During cardiac catheterization, KT received a DES to treat a 90% occlusion of his LAD. In addition to the aspirin he received in the emergency department, which of the following is the most appropriate antiplatelet regimen for KT?
   A. Ticagrelor 180 mg PO × 1; followed by ASA 162 mg PO daily and ticagrelor 90 mg PO bid × 12 months
   B. Ticagrelor 180 mg PO × 1; followed by ASA 81 mg PO daily and ticagrelor 90 mg PO bid × 12 months
   C. Clopidogrel 300 mg PO × 1; followed by ASA 325 mg PO daily and clopidogrel 75 mg PO bid × 12 months
   D. Prasugrel 60 PO × 1; followed by ASA 162 mg PO daily and prasugrel 10 mg PO daily × 6 months

4. Should KT be started on beta-blocker therapy?
   A. Yes, he should be started on a short acting PO beta-blocker like metoprolol tartrate 25 mg PO every 6 hours
   B. Yes, he should be started on a long-acting PO beta blocker like metoprolol succinate 50 mg PO daily
   C. Yes, he should be started on an IV beta-blocker like metoprolol tartrate 5 mg IV q2 min for three doses
   D. No, he should not be started on a beta-blocker as he has a history of DM type 2

5. KT is currently on atorvastatin 20 mg PO daily for lipid management. Should any adjustments be made to this regimen?
   A. Yes, now that the patient has had an ACS, his atorvastatin should be increased to 80 mg PO daily
   B. Yes, now that the patient has had an ACS, he should have ezetimibe 10 mg PO daily added to his therapy
   C. No, moderate intensity statin therapy is appropriate for this patient
   D. No, the patient's AST is elevated, and this could be a side effect related to his statin therapy

6. KT is stable and is now ready to be discharged home. After completing a discharged medication reconciliation, the team will discharge the patient on the following medications:

   Acetaminophen 650 mg PO q6h PRN knee pain
   Aspirin 81 mg PO daily
   Atorvastatin 80 mg PO daily
   HCTZ 25 mg PO daily
   Levothyroxine 88 mcg PO daily

Lisinopril 20 mg PO daily
Metformin ER 1000 mg PO daily
Metoprolol succinate 50 mg PO daily
Multivitamin PO daily
Sertraline 50 mg PO daily
Ticagrelor 90 mg PO bid × 12 months
Nitroglycerin SL 0.4 mg q5min PRN CP

As you go through the discharge medication list with KT, you counsel KT to stop taking ibuprofen and to take acetaminophen instead. What is the reasoning behind discontinuing ibuprofen?

A. Acetaminophen is the first-line therapy for knee pain from osteoarthritis

B. Ibuprofen is contraindicated in patients taking ticagrelor

C. Ibuprofen is contraindicated in post-ACS patients

D. All of the above

7. KT noticed that glucosamine and turmeric was never restarted in the hospital so he wants to know when he could resume these two supplements. What do you tell KT?

A. Glucosamine and turmeric interact with aspirin so KT should stop taking these supplements

B. Glucosamine is safe to resume once the patient is home and it is effective in reducing OA pain; however, KT should stop taking turmeric because it does not provide any health benefits

C. It is safe to resume both supplements once the patient is home

D. Turmeric is safe to resume once the patient is home since it is derived from a plant; however, KT should consider stopping glucosamine because it does not provide any health benefits

8. KT instructs the inpatient team to send the new prescriptions to an independent pharmacy where he regularly fills his prescriptions. Upon final verification of ticagrelor, a DUR pops up, indicating there is a drug–drug interaction with an SSRI. Which of the following statements best describe the drug–drug interaction and the appropriate follow-up plan?

A. Sertraline may decrease the levels of ticagrelor, the community pharmacist should call the hospitalist to change the sertraline to another antidepressant in a different class

B. Sertraline may enhance the antiplatelet effect of ticagrelor, the community pharmacist should instruct the patient to monitor for signs and symptoms of bleeding

C. Ticagrelor may decrease the effectiveness of sertraline, the community pharmacist should call the hospitalist to change ticagrelor to a different antiplatelet that does not cause the same drug–drug interaction

D. Ticagrelor may inhibit the metabolism of sertraline, the community pharmacist should instruct the patient to monitor for signs and symptoms of serotonin syndrome

9. KT presents to his primary care office a week after discharged for a post-hospitalization follow-up. At the follow-up appointment, KT complained that he has too many pills and wanted to know if there is a way to streamline his medications. Which of the following option(s) would be appropriate?

i. Consider discontinuing HCTZ; however, increase the dose of lisinopril to maintain adequate blood pressure control

ii. Consider discontinuing lisinopril; however, increase the dose of HCTZ to maintain adequate blood pressure control

iii. Consider switching lisinopril and HCTZ to a combination product

A. i and ii

B. ii and iii

C. i and iii

D. All of the above

REFERENCES

1. Amsterdam EA, Wenger NK, Brindis RG, et al. 2014 AHA/ACC guideline for the management of patients with non–ST-elevation acute coronary syndromes. *J Am Coll Cardiol.* 2014;64(24):e139-e228.

2. Grundy SM, Stone NJ, Bailey AL, et al. 2018 AHA/ACC/AACVPR/AAPA/ ABC/ACPM/ADA/AGS/APhA/ASPC/NLA/PCNA guideline on the management of blood cholesterol. *J Am Coll Cardiol.* 2019;73(24):e285-e350.

3. Kolasinski SL, Neogi T, Hochberg MC, et al. 2019 American College of Rheumatology/Arthritis Foundation Guideline for the Management of Osteoarthritis of the Hand, Hip, and Knee. *Arthritis Care Res.* 2020;72(2):149-162.

15 Heart Failure with Reduced Ejection Fraction

Elizabeth A. Cook   Jessica Wooster

PATIENT PRESENTATION

Chief Complaint

"I'm breathing more easily and my legs are much less swollen."

History of Present Illness

AK is a 52-year-old white male newly diagnosed with heart failure with reduced ejection fraction (HFrEF) after presenting to the emergency department to evaluate dyspnea that has increased in severity over approximately 5 days. AK had noted dyspnea on exertion when performing routine activities of daily living, three-pillow orthopnea, nonproductive cough accompanied by general malaise, 4 kg weight gain, and +2 bilateral pitting edema with diminished pedal pulses upon presentation. He denied fever, chest pain, and hemoptysis. Additionally, he denied abdominal pain, nausea/vomiting, or diarrhea.

AK was subsequently admitted to a telemetry unit. His brain natriuretic peptide (BNP) was noted to be severely elevated (1305 pg/mL) and echocardiogram revealed left ventricular dysfunction with ejection fraction (EF) 25% to 30%. He was aggressively diuresed per protocol to dry weight. After a total of 3 days of acute care, he has stabilized with disposition to discharge home to self-care.

Past Medical History

Type 2 diabetes mellitus (T2DM)
Hypertension (HTN)
Hyperlipidemia (HLD)
Coronary artery disease (CAD)
Myocardial infarction (MI) in 2017

Surgical History

Placement of drug-eluting stents (DES) × 3 in 2017

Family History

Father: CAD
Mother: T2DM

Social History

Widowed, retired school maintenance supervisor.
Lives independently but has three children who are supportive and visit frequently.
Denies tobacco use.
Drinks 4 to 5 alcoholic beverages on weekends.

Immunization

Up to date

Insurance

Medicaid

Allergies

No known drug allergies

Home Medications Prior to Admission

- Aspirin 81 mg PO daily
- Dapagliflozin 10 mg PO daily
- Lisinopril 10 mg PO daily
- Metformin 1000 mg PO bid
- Nitroglycerin 0.4 mg SL PRN chest pain (CP). May repeat in 5 minutes if CP does not subside. Do not exceed 3 tablets in 15 minutes.
- Propranolol 40 mg PO bid
- Rosiglitazone 4 mg PO daily
- Semaglutide 0.5 mg SQ q week
- Simvastatin 20 mg PO qHS

Inpatient Medications

- Aspirin 81 mg PO daily
- Insulin aspart per sliding scale
- Furosemide 20 mg PO daily
- Lisinopril 10 mg PO daily

- Nitroglycerin 0.4 mg SL PRN CP. May repeat in 5 minutes if CP does not subside. Do not exceed 3 tablets in 15 minutes.
- Propranolol 40 mg PO bid
- Atorvastatin 10 mg PO qHS

Physical Examination

▶ Vital Signs

Temp 37°C, P 85, RR: 25, BP 142/98 mmHg, pO_2 92%, Ht: 5'8", Wt: 79 kg

▶ General

Patient sitting up on hospital bed in no apparent distress.

▶ Neurologic

A&O × 3.

▶ HEENT

PERRLA.

▶ Neck

JVD (−), carotid bruit not appreciated.

▶ Respiratory

Wheezes (−), mild crackles noted in both lung fields, but improved from admission.

▶ Cardiovascular

Rate and rhythm unremarkable upon auscultation.

▶ Abdomen

Soft, nontender, nondistended, hyperactive bowel sounds.

▶ Skin

Warm, pink, moist.

▶ Extremities

+1 pitting pedal edema bilaterally; radial and pedal pulses evident.

Laboratory Values

Na = 136 mEq/L	HbA1c = 6.2%
K = 2.9 mEq/L	TC = 126 mg/dL
Cl = 100 mEq/L	LDL = 135 mg/dL
CO_2 = 27 mEq/L	HDL = 38 mg/dL
BUN = 10 mg/dL	TG = 98 mg/dL
SCr = 0.9 mg/dL	BNP = 258 pg/mL
Glu = 106 mg/dL	
Ca = 9 mg/dL	
Mg = 2.2 mg/dL	

Diagnostic Tests

▶ Chest X-Ray

One PA view chest radiograph was obtained and shows signs of potential interstitial pulmonary edema including enlarged and loss of definition of large pulmonary vessels, both Kerley's A and Kerley's B lines associated with cardiomegaly. Findings suggest bilateral pulmonary vascular congestion with mild interstitial edema.

▶ Electrocardiogram

Normal sinus rhythm (NSR)

▶ Echocardiogram

EF 25%−30%

QUESTIONS

1. Which of AK's home medications carries the greatest potential to exacerbate his newly diagnosed HFrEF if it is restarted upon discharge?
   A. Dapagliflozin
   B. Metformin
   C. Rosiglitazone
   D. Semaglutide

2. Your medical team is evaluating AK's beta-blocker therapy prior to discharge to determine if changes are necessary. Which of the following is the most appropriate recommendation?
   A. Continue propranolol at 40 mg PO bid
   B. Change propranolol to metoprolol tartrate 12.5 mg PO bid
   C. Changed propranolol to carvedilol 50 mg PO bid
   D. Change propranolol to bisoprolol 5 mg PO qd

3. As a newly diagnosed HF patient, AK requires self-management education to reduce his likelihood of hospital readmission. Which of the following statements provides AK with the most accurate medical advice?
   A. Limit dietary sodium intake to <5 g per day
   B. Restrict fluid intake to <0.5 L per day
   C. Contact your healthcare provider if you experience >5-pound weight gain in 1 week
   D. Avoid physical activity to reduce likelihood of symptom exacerbation

4. Your medical team would like to minimize CV risk factors to prevent future events that could worsen HF and are seeking advice on how to best manage AK's lipids prior to discharge. Which of the following is the best clinical recommendation?
   A. Continue atorvastatin 10 mg PO qHS
   B. Increase atorvastatin from 10 mg to 40 mg PO qHS
   C. Continue atorvastatin 10 mg PO qHS and add ezetimibe 10 mg PO daily
   D. Continue atorvastatin 10 mg PO qHS and add alirocumab 75 mg SQ every 2 weeks

5. Upon review of predischarge labs, your medical team plans to initiate potassium chloride supplementation, as AK is

experiencing mild hypokalemia. Which of his newly initiated/adjusted medications is most likely contributing to this condition?

A. Lisinopril

B. Insulin aspart

C. Furosemide

D. Atorvastatin

6. AK presents to his outpatient cardiologist's clinic 7 days after hospital discharge for follow-up. Per his discharge summary, you see his HFrEF regimen consists of the following: furosemide 20 mg PO daily, lisinopril 20 mg PO daily, potassium chloride 10 mEq PO daily, and bisoprolol 5 mg PO daily. He attests to taking all home medications as prescribed. AK mentions that it was recommended by the medical team at hospital discharge that he start sacubitril/valsartan for his HFrEF, as it is the preferred agent over lisinopril, but they did not start it before discharge. You agree with the discharge medical team and plan to start sacubitril/valsartan in the patient. When should AK initiate his newly provisioned sacubitril/valsartan therapy?

A. Immediately, use in conjunction with lisinopril augments therapeutic effects

B. Twenty-four hours after discontinuing lisinopril

C. Thirty-six hours after discontinuing lisinopril

D. During his next hospitalization to ensure appropriate monitoring

7. AK presents to his outpatient cardiologist's clinic 7 days after hospital discharge for follow-up. His vital signs today are as follows: Height: 5'8", Weight: 78 kg, blood pressure: 140/92 mmHg, heart rate: 72 bpm. Pertinent laboratory values obtained at this visit include SCr: 1.1 mg/dL, eGFR: >60 mL/min/1.73 m2, Na: 137 mmol/L, K: 4.2 mmol/L. Based on AK's medication regimen, vital signs, and laboratory results, which of the following would be an appropriate starting dose of sacubitril/valsartan?

A. Sacubitril 24 mg/valsartan 26 mg PO bid

B. Sacubitril 49 mg/valsartan 51 mg PO bid

C. Sacubitril 97 mg/valsartan 103 mg PO bid

D. Sacubitril/valsartan contraindicated based on laboratory parameters and vital signs

8. AK informs your team that he has Medicaid insurance and is concerned that his new prescription for sacubitril/valsartan will be costly. Which of the following is the best recommendation for AK to ensure long-term adherence to sacubitril/valsartan?

A. Indefinitely supply AK with free sacubitril/valsartan samples from clinic

B. Initiate prior authorization paperwork to ensure AK's medication is covered by insurance

C. Enroll AK in the drug manufacturer's patient assistance program

D. Provide AK with a 30-day free trial coupon each month

9. Which of the following adverse effects should AK be monitored for following initiation of sacubitril/valsartan?

A. Hypotension, hyperkalemia, increased serum creatinine, cough

B. Hypertension, hyperkalemia, increased serum creatinine, cough

C. Hypotension, hypokalemia, decreased serum creatinine, cough

D. Hypertension, hypokalemia, decreased serum creatinine, cough

REFERENCES

1. U.S. Department of Health and Human Services Food and Drug Administration, Center for Drug Evaluation and Research Guidance for Industry. Diabetes Mellitus: Evaluating Cardiovascular Risk in New Antidiabetic Therapies to Treat Type 2 Diabetes. 2008:1-5. FDA, Maryland.

2. Pagell RL, O'Bryant CL, Cheng D, Chow TJ, et al. Drugs that may cause or exacerbate heart failure. *Circulation*. 2016;134:e32-e69.

3. The American Diabetes Association. Cardiovascular disease and risk management: standards of medical care in diabetes 2020. *Diabetes Care*. 2020;43(suppl 1):S111-S134.

4. Yancy CW, Jessup M, Bozkurt B, Butler J, et al. 2013 ACCF/AHA guideline for the management of heart failure: a report of the American College of Cardiology Foundation/American Heart Association Task Force on Practice Guidelines. *J Am Coll Cardiol*. 2013;62(16):e147-e239.

5. Yancy CW, Jessup M, Bozkurt B, et al. 2017 ACC/AHA/HFSA focused update of the 2013 ACCF/AHA guideline for the management of heart failure: a report of the American College of Cardiology/American Heart Association Task Force on Clinical Practice Guidelines and the Heart Failure Society of America. *Circulation*. 2017;136(6):e137.

6. Doukky R, Avery E, Mangla A, et al. Impact of dietary sodium restriction on heart failure outcomes. *JACC Heart Fail*. 2016;4(1):24-35.

7. Castro-Gutiérrez V, Rada G. Is fluid restriction needed in heart failure? *Medwave*. 2017;17(suppl 1):e6817.

8. Taylor RS, Sagar VA, Davies EJ, Briscoe S, et al. Exercise-based rehabilitation for heart failure. *Cochrane Database Syst Rev*. 2014(4):CD003331.

9. Grundy SM, Stone NJ, Bailey AL, et al. 2018 AHA/ACC/AACVPR/AAPA/ABC/ACPM/ADA/AGS/APhA/ASPC/NLA/PCNA guideline on the management of blood cholesterol: a report of the American College of Cardiology/American Heart Association Task Force on Clinical Practice Guidelines [published correction appears in *J Am Coll Cardiol*. 2019 Jun 25;73(24):3237-3241.] *J Am Coll Cardiol*. 2019;73(24):e285.

10. Entresto (sacubitril/valsartan) tablets [package insert]. East Hanover, NJ: Novartis Pharmaceuticals Corp.; October 2019.

11. Senni M, McMurray JJV, Wachter R, et al. Initiating sacubitril/valsartan (LCZ696) in heart failure: results of TITRATION, a double-blind, randomized comparison of two uptitration regimens. *Eur J Heart Fail*. 2016;18(9):1193-1202.

16 Atrial Fibrillation and Stroke Prevention

Laura Tsu   Laressa Bethishou

PATIENT PRESENTATION

Chief Complaint

Chest pain and difficulty breathing

History of Present Illness and Hospital Course

RE is a 70-year-old Hispanic female who has been treated for atrial fibrillation (AF) with rapid ventricular response (RVR). She was initially brought in by ambulance for chest pain and shortness of breath. After a myocardial infarction (MI) was ruled out, she was treated for AF with RVR. She is recovering on the telemetry floor and the medical team is planning to discharge her later today. She has trouble with keeping her INR within range and she complains about needing to get too many labs.

Past Medical History

Hypertension
Type 2 diabetes
Heart failure
Atrial fibrillation
Stroke 2 years ago

Surgical History

Hysterectomy

Family History

Mother: had two heart attacks and died of heart failure at age 73
Father: had hypertension and died at age 79 after an MI

Social History

The patient lives with her daughter, using a walker to ambulate through her home.

She denies smoking for the past 20 years but used to smoke 1 pack per day × 25 years prior to that. She denies any alcohol use.

Patient is Spanish speaking.

Allergies

No known drug allergies

Immunization

Up to date

Insurance

Aetna Medicare Advantage

Home Medications

- Metformin XR 750 mg PO bid
- Insulin glargine U-100 SC 28 units nightly
- Lisinopril 5 mg PO daily
- Atenolol 25 mg PO daily
- Furosemide 20 mg PO daily
- Warfarin 4 mg PO MWF, 2 mg PO Tu/Th/Sat/Sun
- MVI 1 tab PO daily
- NTG 0.4 mg SL PRN chest pain

Inpatient Medications

- Insulin lispro SC sliding scale
- Warfarin 4 mg PO MWF, 2 mg PO Tu/Th/Sat/Sun
- Furosemide 40 mg PO daily
- Lisinopril 5 mg PO daily
- Metoprolol tartrate 25 mg PO bid
- Atorvastatin 20 mg PO daily
- MVI, 1 tab PO daily
- NTG 0.4 mg SL PRN chest pain
- Docusate sodium 100 mg PO twice daily PRN for constipation

Physical Examination

▶ Vital Signs

BP 128/78 mmHg, P 72; RR 16; Temp 98.8°F; Ht: 61″, Wt: 95 kg

▶ General

Obese Hispanic female, resting comfortably, A&O × 4.

▶ HEENT

Normocephalic, PERRLA, mild JVD, supple, no lymphadenopathy.

▶ Cardiovascular

S1/S2, no murmurs.

▶ Pulmonary

RLL and LLL dull to percussion posteriorly.

▶ Abdominal

Soft; nontender/nondistended; normoactive bowel sounds.

▶ Genitourinary

Normal female genitalia.

▶ Extremities

Radial pulses 1+ bilaterally, pedal pulses 1+ bilaterally, extremities warm and well-perfused.

Laboratory Findings

▶ CMP

Lab	Results
Na^+	140
K^+	4.5
Cl^-	105
HCO_3^-	20
Creatinine	1.1
CrCl	71
BUN	20
Glucose	138
Ca^{2+}	8.2
Phosphorous	4.3
Magnesium	2.1

▶ CBC

Lab	Results
WBC	4.0×10^3 cells/L
Hgb	11 g/dL
Hct	25.4%
Platelets	200×10^9

▶ Lipids

Lab	Results
Total cholesterol	220
Triglycerides	126
HDL	35
LDL	160

▶ Other

Lab	Results
AST	20
ALT	28
Alk Phos	55
Albumin	4.1
NT-BNP	865
A1c	8.9%
aPTT	40
INR	1.5

Diagnostic Tests

▶ Chest X-Ray

Mild pulmonary edema and cardiomegaly

▶ Electrocardiogram

Atrial fibrillation with no p waves, QTc 449 ms

▶ Echocardiogram

EF 25%–30%, left ventricle appears dilated, moderate hypokinesis of the inferior and anterior wall

QUESTIONS

1. Which factor could have contributed to RE's fluctuating INR readings?
   A. Inconsistent diet of vitamin K-containing foods
   B. Drug interaction with multivitamin
   C. Taking warfarin at different times of the day
   D. Inconsistent exercise routines

2. What is RE's CHA_2DS_2-VASc score?
   A. 5
   B. 6
   C. 7
   D. 8

3. Which antithrombotic therapy would be the best option for RE?
   A. Rivaroxaban 20 mg PO daily
   B. Aspirin 81 mg PO daily
   C. Enoxaparin 100 mg SC bid
   D. Apixaban 10 mg PO bid for 7 days, then 5 mg PO bid

4. Which counseling point for direct oral anticoagulants is accurate?
   A. Discard edoxaban 120 days after opening the container
   B. Take rivaroxaban with your evening meal
   C. Keep a consistent intake of green leafy vegetables with dabigatran
   D. Keep apixaban in its original container

5. Which beta-blocker would be the best option for RE?
   A. Atenolol 25 mg PO daily
   B. Metoprolol tartrate 25 mg PO bid
   C. Metoprolol succinate 50 mg PO daily
   D. Propranolol 80 mg PO daily

6. Would amiodarone be a good recommendation for RE?
   A. Yes, it is beneficial for patients with heart failure and atrial fibrillation.
   B. Yes, it is preferred to help control RE's heart rate.
   C. No, there is a drug interaction with warfarin.
   D. No, a beta-blocker is preferred for rate control.

7. What is the best recommendation regarding RE's statin therapy?
   A. Change to rosuvastatin 40 mg daily
   B. Change to simvastatin 80 mg daily
   C. Discontinue atorvastatin and start ezetimibe
   D. Continue current therapy of atorvastatin 20 mg daily

8. Which monitoring test is most important for RE's rivaroxaban therapy in 3 to 6 months?
   A. Basic metabolic panel
   B. INR
   C. Liver function tests
   D. Pulmonary function tests

9. Which of the following medications should be continued on discharge?
   A. Metformin XR 750 mg PO bid
   B. Atenolol 25 mg daily
   C. Warfarin 4 mg PO MWF, 2 mg PO Tu/Th/Sat/Sun
   D. All of the above

10. Comprehensive discharge planning for this patient should include which of the following:
    A. Sending her new prescriptions to the pharmacy to confirm coverage
    B. Coordinating discharge education with an interpreter
    C. Engaging the patient and family/caregivers
    D. All of the above

REFERENCES

1. January CT, Wann LS, Calkins H, et al. 2019 AHA/ACC/HRS focused update of the 2014 AHA/ACC/HRS guideline for the management of patients with atrial fibrillation: a report of the American College of Cardiology/American Heart Association Task Force on Clinical Practice Guidelines and the Heart Rhythm Society in Collaboration with the Society of Thoracic Surgeons. *Circulation.* 2019;140(2):125-151.

2. Lip GYH, Banerjee A, Boriani G, et al. Antithrombotic therapy for atrial fibrillation: CHEST Guideline and Expert Panel Report. *Chest.* 2018;154(5):1121-1201.

3. Wyse DG, Waldo AL, DiMarco JP, et al. A comparison of rate control and rhythm control in patients with atrial fibrillation. *N Engl J Med.* 2002;347(23):1825-1833.

4. Amarenco P, Bogousslavsky J, Callahan A 3rd, et al. High-dose atorvastatin after stroke or transient ischemic attack [published correction appears in *N Engl J Med.* 2018 Jun 13;null]. *N Engl J Med.* 2006;355(6):549-559.

Section 5

Patients with Respiratory Conditions

17 Optimizing Asthma Therapy Through the Continuum of Care

Luma Munjy

Jeffrey Gonzales

Laressa Bethishou

PATIENT PRESENTATION

Chief Complaint

JR is a 23-year-old female who is being discharged from the hospital following a severe asthma exacerbation. She requires adjustment of her asthma medications to prevent a future exacerbation.

History of Present Illness

JR presented to the emergency department 3 days ago in acute respiratory distress with increased work of breathing and inspiratory and expiratory wheeze. It was determined that JR was having a moderate-severe asthma exacerbation due to uncontrolled asthma. Prior to admission, JR was recovering from a viral upper respiratory tract infection and started to have difficulty breathing during soccer practice for her college soccer team. JR used her albuterol rescue inhaler several times without relief and finally was brought to the emergency department by her coach.

Past Medical History

Type I diabetes mellitus
Allergic rhinitis
Atopic dermatitis
Asthma
Achilles tendonitis
Acute stage fright

Social History

College student in final year of studies to become a teacher.
Plays for the college soccer team.
Denies illicit drug use, smoking, or alcohol use.

Allergies

Aspirin (hives)

Immunization

Vaccine	Up to date
Tdap	Yes
Varicella	Yes
HPV	Yes
MenACWY	Yes
MenB	Yes
MMR	Yes

Insurance

Aetna HMO

Home Medications

- Albuterol HFA MDI: 90 mcg 1–2 puffs every 4–6 hours PRN shortness of breath/wheezing
- Beclomethasone HFA MDI: 80 mcg: 1 puff inhaled twice daily
- Cetirizine 10 mg PO once daily
- Montelukast 10 mg PO once daily
- Ibuprofen 200 mg PO every 6 hours for Achilles tendonitis
- Propranolol 10 mg PO 1 hour prior to event for acute stage fright
- Lantus 20 units SQ once daily
- Humalog per sliding scale: 20 units SQ for every 15 grams of carbohydrates
- Hydrocortisone 1% cream: apply a thin film to affected area 2 times daily

Inpatient Medications

- Ipratropium 0.5 mg/albuterol solution: oral inhalation via nebulizer every 20 minutes for 3 doses

- Methylprednisolone 125 mg IV X1 dose
- Oxygen to achieve $SaO_2 \geq 90\%$

Physical Examination

▶ *Vital Signs*

BP 118/73 mmHg, HR 75 bpm, RR 18, O_2 saturation: 98%, Ht: 5'7", Wt: 140 lbs

▶ *General*

Well developed, well-nourished Hispanic female in mild respiratory distress.

▶ *HEENT*

Red, watery eyes. Throat appears red with slight swelling.

▶ *Chest*

Mild sibilant rhonchi (wheezing).

▶ *Cardiovascular*

RRR, S1, and S2 normal, no rubs, gallops, or murmurs.

Laboratory Findings

WBC	18,800 cells/mL
Neutrophils	11,840 cells/mL
Lymphocytes	4,320 cells/mL
Monocytes	750 cells/mL
Basophils	760 cells/mL
Eosinophils	1,130 cells/mL

Diagnostic Tests

▶ *Chest X-Ray*

Normal lung fields, no infiltrates

▶ *Electrocardiogram*

Sinus tachycardia

QUESTIONS

1. Which of the following statements, provided when interviewing the patient on admission, is indicative of an adherence barrier?
   A. "I occasionally forget to take my cetirizine"
   B. "I'm not sure what an asthma action plan is"
   C. "I don't always pick up my inhaler due to cost"
   D. "My albuterol inhaler is what makes me feel better"
   E. All of the above

2. Which of JR's home medications could be contributing to the severity of her asthma exacerbation?
   A. Lantus and ibuprofen
   B. Ibuprofen and propranolol
   C. Propranolol and montelukast
   D. Humalog and cetirizine

3. It is determined that the patient is currently at step 3 according to the GINA step therapy chart and that she needs to be stepped up one step. What is the most appropriate medication for treatment based on current GINA guidelines?
   A. Beclomethasone HFA MDI 80 mcg: 2 puffs bid
   B. Budesonide/formoterol 160 mcg/4.5 mcg MDI: 2 puffs bid and 1 puff PRN SOB
   C. Budesonide/formoterol 160 mcg/4.5 mcg MDI: 1 puff bid and 1 puff PRN SOB
   D. Beclomethasone HFA MDI 80 mcg: 1 puff bid plus 2 puffs of albuterol HFA 90 mcg/actuation whenever ICS inhaler is used

4. JR admits she does not always use her beclomethasone MDI as it does not work as well as her albuterol. Which of the following counseling points are important when educating this patient?
   A. It is okay to keep using albuterol as long as it is helping
   B. Not being adherent to beclomethasone MDI can lead to more frequent exacerbations, necessitating the use of oral glucocorticosteroids, leading to less blood sugar control
   C. It may take 1 to 2 weeks to see the benefit of inhaled corticosteroids
   D. All of the above

5. Which of the following interventions should be included in comprehensive discharge planning for our patient?
   A. Our patient should receive appropriate vaccinations including influenza and pneumococcal conjugate
   B. The patient should be educated to contact her physician and provide a summary of her hospitalization
   C. Her prescriptions should be sent to her pharmacy in advance of hospital discharge to ensure coverage
   D. All of the above

6. Based on JR's vaccination history and comorbidities, what vaccine(s) should JR receive prior to discharge?
   A. Pneumococcal polysaccharide and influenza
   B. Pneumococcal conjugate and influenza
   C. Influenza only
   D. Vaccinations are up to date

7. Three weeks later, JR presents to the clinic for follow-up stating she feels her maintenance therapy for her asthma is not working. What is the most appropriate action?
   A. Evaluate inhaler technique
   B. Increase her inhaler therapy
   C. Consider adding omalizumab
   D. No action at this time as it is too soon

8. Which of the following represents proper use of an MDI?
   A. Inhaler should be shaken well prior to use. Remove dust cap from mouthpiece of inhaler. Breath out completely. Place lips around the mouthpiece. Breath in slowly and completely while pressing down on the top of the inhaler canister to activate the inhaler. Hold your breath for 10 seconds to allow the medication to reach the airways in the lungs.

B. Inhaler should be shaken well prior to use. Remove dust cap from mouthpiece of inhaler. Breath out completely. Place lips around the mouthpiece. Breath in hard and fast while pressing down on the top of the inhaler canister to activate the inhaler. Hold your breath for 10 seconds to allow the medication to reach the airways in the lungs.

C. Inhaler should be shaken well prior to use. Remove dust cap from mouthpiece of inhaler. Breath in. Place lips around the mouthpiece. Breath in slowly and completely while pressing down on the top of the inhaler canister to activate the inhaler. Hold your breath for 10 seconds to allow the medication to reach the airways in the lungs.

D. Inhaler should be shaken well prior to use. Remove dust cap from mouthpiece of inhaler. Breath out completely. Place lips around the mouthpiece. Breath in slowly and completely while pressing down on the top of the inhaler canister to activate the inhaler. Hold your breath for 1 minute to allow the medication to reach the airways in the lungs.

9. It has now been 6 weeks since JR has been on her new dose of medium dose ICS/LABA for both control and relief of symptoms. She presents to her outpatient clinic for follow-up. Her symptoms are now under control and she reports that she does not require use of her inhaler to relieve symptoms of asthma, she has no nighttime awakenings, and she has no limitations of daily activity. Her lung function is assessed through a peak flow meter and it is noted that her peak expiratory flow is >80%. How should her asthma therapy be managed at this time?

A. Step up one step

B. Maintain current step

C. Step down one step

D. Step down two steps

10. You receive a phone call from your patient. The patient is irate. She has just gone to pick up a refill on her ICS/LABA MDI and was told it would cost $400. It is not covered by her prescription insurance. Her pharmacist states it is 7 days too soon to fill. The patient states she has been using 2 puffs twice a day plus 2 puffs when she is short of breath. What should be done to help resolve the situation and ensure your patient has access to medication therapy?

A. Inform the patient she must pay out of pocket for the prescription if she wants the medication.

B. This patient's asthma is not well controlled. Contact her provider and recommend a step up in their asthma therapy.

C. Recommend to the patient's provider they provide a prescription for an inhaler containing an equivalent dose of their ICS only and a SABA inhaler. Instruct the patient to use 2 puffs of each inhaler bid and PRN SOB.

D. Recommend to the patient's provider to add long-term OCS to the patient's therapy.

REFERENCES

1. Global Initiative for Asthma. Global Strategy for Asthma Management and Prevention. 2020 Update. Available at https://ginasthma.org/. Accessed May 31, 2020.

2. Centers for Disease Control and Prevention. Recommended Adult Immunization Schedule for ages 19 years or older, United States, 2020. Available at https://www.cdc.gov/vaccines/schedules/hcp/imz/adult.html. Accessed May 31, 2020.

18 Managing Pneumonia in Chronic Obstructive Lung Disease

Rupal Mansukhani

PATIENT PRESENTATION

Chief Complaint

"I am having trouble breathing."

History of Present Illness

RM is a 64-year-old male who comes to the emergency department with fever, shortness of breath, and cough. He complains of a productive cough with discolored sputum for the past week. Over the past few days, he complains of fever, chills, and pressure on his chest when he coughs. He has been hospitalized two times in the past year approximately 6 months ago for COPD exacerbation.

Past Medical History

Chronic obstructive pulmonary disease (COPD)
Diabetes type II
Hypertension (HTN)

Surgical History

N/A

Family History

Father: had COPD and HTN and passed away from a stroke
Mother: is 88 y/o, alive, with coronary artery disease

Social History

He lives alone, never married.
He smokes 1 pack per day for 30 years. He quit 5 years ago.
He drinks beer occasionally, 1 to 2 times per month.

Immunization

Up to date

Insurance

United Healthcare

Allergies

No known drug allergies

Home Medications

- Anoro Ellipta 62.5 mcg/25 mcg: 1 puff daily
- Albuterol metered-dose inhaler: 2 puffs every 4 hours as needed for shortness of breath
- Lisinopril 10 mg PO daily
- Metformin 1000 mg PO twice daily

Physical Examination

▶ **Vital Signs**

Temp 101.5°F, P 128, RR 24, BP 118/78 mmHg, SpO_2 70%, Ht: 5′6″, Wt: 72.7 kg

▶ **General**

Chronically ill-appearing male with shortness of breath in moderate distress.

▶ **HEENT**

Normocephalic, atraumatic, PERRLA, EOMI.

▶ **Pulmonary**

Diminished breath sounds and crackles bilaterally.

▶ **Cardiovascular**

NSR, no m/r/g.

▶ **Abdomen**

Soft, non-distended, nontender.

▶ **Genitourinary**

Normal male genitalia, no complaints of dysuria, or hematuria.

▶ **Neurologic**

Awake, alert.

▶ **Extremities**

No edema.

Laboratory Findings

Na 137 mEq/L	RBC 3.8 × 106/mm³	WBC 23.1 × 103/mm³	Procalcitonin 1.9 ng/mL
K 4.1 mEq/L	Hgb 12.1 g/dL	Neutrophils 67%	Lactic acid 2.3 mmol/L
Cl 103 mEq/L	Hct 35%	Bands 15%	
CO_2 27 mEq/L	MCV 91 μm³	Lymphs 12%	
BUN 42 mg/dL	MCHC 35 g/dL	Monos 6%	
SCr 1.4 mg/dL	Plt 220 × 103/mm³	Eosinophils 400 cells/uL	
Glu 260 mg/dL			

Diagnostic Tests

▶ **CAT score**

22

▶ **CT Chest**

The heart size is normal. There is consolidation of the right lower lobe and lateral segment of the middle lobe, with air bronchograms likely pneumonia. The left lung is clear. No pleural effusions.

▶ **Blood Cultures**

Pending.

QUESTIONS

1. Which laboratory test(s) help identify if a patient needs treatment for pneumonia?
   A. Procalcitonin 1.9 ng/mL
   B. WBC 23.1 × 103/mm³
   C. Chest imaging
   D. All of the above

2. Based on the GOLD guidelines, what cardinal symptom must you have to start empiric treatment of antibiotics?
   A. Dyspnea
   B. Sputum volume
   C. Sputum purulence
   D. Fever

3. When choosing an antibiotic, what pathogens should be covered?
   A. *Streptococcus pneumoniae*
   B. *Haemophilus influenzae*
   C. Atypical bacteria such as *Mycoplasma pneumoniae*
   D. All of the above

4. Which of the following classes of medication is preferred for acute exacerbations?
   A. Short-acting bronchodilators
   B. Inhaled corticosteroid
   C. Long-acting inhaled beta2-agonist
   D. Long-acting anticholinergic

5. What are the main treatment goals for COPD?
   A. Complete remission of the disease
   B. Reducing the risk of exacerbation
   C. Helping patients with end-of-life care
   D. Optimizing functions

6. In the inpatient setting, which antibiotic regimen is most appropriate for treatment of community-acquired pneumonia (CAP)?
   A. Beta-lactam
   B. Macrolide
   C. Beta-lactam plus vancomycin
   D. Beta-lactam plus macrolide

7. If a patient is started with prednisone therapy, which dose and duration is most appropriate?
   A. Prednisone 20 mg daily for 10 days
   B. Prednisone 40 mg daily for 5 days
   C. Prednisone 80 mg daily for 10 days
   D. Prednisone 120 mg daily for 5 days

8. At discharge, what pharmacologic therapy is most appropriate for the management of COPD in this patient?
   A. LABA
   B. LAMA
   C. LABA + LAMA
   D. LABA + LAMA + ICS

REFERENCE

1. Global Initiative for Chronic Obstructive Lung Disease Global strategy for the diagnosis, management and prevention of chronic obstructive pulmonary disease (2020). Available at https://goldcopd.org/wp-content/uploads/2019/11/GOLD-2020-REPORT-ver1.0wms.pdf. Accessed July 30, 2020.

Section 6

Special Populations

19 Care Considerations in the Elderly

Tianrui Yang   Jessica Wooster

PATIENT PRESENTATION

Chief Complaint

"I feel dizzy and out of it."

History of Present Illness

WL is an 82-year-old Caucasian female brought to the emergency department by her daughter after finding her mother to be very lethargic and weak. Patient states that she has been feeling tired and out of it all the time lately, so she stays in bed a lot. When she tried to get up from the bed, she felt like she was going to faint and had to sit back down for a minute before trying to get up again. Upon questioning, she also states that she fell a couple of times in the past month but luckily didn't break anything, so she did not come to the emergency room. She states that she has chronic back pain but currently she is only experiencing stiffness and no pain.

Past Medical History

Hypertension (HTN)
Heart failure with reduced ejection fraction (HFrEF)
Generalized anxiety disorder
Type 2 diabetes mellitus (DM)
Neuropathy
Chronic back pain
Chronic kidney disease (CKD)
Seasonal allergies

Surgical History

Appendectomy, cesarean section

Family History

Father: had CAD and passed away from a myocardial infarction at age 50
Mother: has type 2 DM and hypothyroidism

Social History

Since her husband passed away 4 years ago, she has been living alone.
Son and daughter live about 1.5 hours away and visit their mother every other week to check in on her.
Drinks alcohol occasionally (3–4 times per month).
Does not smoke or use illicit drugs.

Immunization

All immunizations up to date

Insurance

Medicare

Allergies

No known drug allergies

Home Medications

- Sacubitril/valsartan 97/103 mg PO bid (started 2 years ago)
- Carvedilol 25 mg PO bid (started 8 years ago)
- Spironolactone 50 mg PO daily (started 5 years ago)
- Furosemide 40 mg PO daily (started 8 years ago)
- Clonidine 0.2 mg PO bid (started 20 years ago)
- Gabapentin 300 mg PO tid (started 15 years ago)
- Hydrocodone/acetaminophen 10/325 mg PO q6h PRN pain (started 20 years ago, takes about 1 to 2 times daily)
- Trazodone 100 mg qHS (started 6 months ago)
- Alprazolam 1 mg PO tid (started 30 years ago at a lower dose)
- Diphenhydramine 25 mg PO daily PRN allergy (started 50 years ago)
- Ergocalciferol 1000 units PO daily (started 20 years ago)
- Calcium carbonate 600 mg PO daily (started 20 years ago)

- Multivitamin 1 tablet PO daily (started 50 years ago)
- Metformin 1 g PO bid (started 40 years ago)
- Empagliflozin 25 mg PO daily (started 3 years ago)

Physical Examination

▶ Vital Signs

Temp 99°F, P 54, RR 24, BP 92/68 mmHg, pO$_2$ 92% Ht: 5′2″, Wt: 50 kg

▶ General

Frail female. Appears weak and sedated.

▶ HEENT

Normocephalic, atraumatic, PERRLA, EOMI, normal fundoscopic exam, normal visual fields.

▶ Pulmonary

Mild rales can be heard.

▶ Cardiovascular

Bradycardic, no m/r/g.

▶ Abdomen

Soft, non-distended, nontender, normal bowel sounds.

▶ Genitourinary

Deferred. No complaints of dysuria or hematuria.

▶ Neurologic

Lethargic and sedated, oriented to place, person, and time when woken up but hard to arouse.

▶ Extremities

No cyanosis or clubbing. 1+ pitting edema in the lower extremity.

Laboratory Findings

Na 136 mEq/L	Ca 8.2 mg/dL	WBC 7.3 × 10^3/μL
K 3.7 mEq/L	Mg 2.1 mg/dL	Hgb 12.7 g/dL
Cl 103 mEq/L	PO$_4$ 4.1 mg/dL	Hct 38%
HCO$_3$ 26 mEq/L	AST 22 U/L	Plt 256 × 10^3/μL
BUN 19 mg/dL	ALT 15 U/L	
SCr 1.5 mg/dL	T Bili 0.9 mg/dL	
Glu 130 mg/dL	Alk Phos 81 U/L	
A1c 6.8%	eGFR 36 mL/ minute/1.73m²	

Diagnostic Tests

▶ Echocardiogram

The left ventricle is moderately dilated. There is normal left ventricular wall thickness. Left ventricular systolic function is moderately reduced. Ejection fraction = 25%–30%. There is moderate anterior wall hypokinesis.

Right ventricle: moderately dilated; normal right ventricular wall thickness; right ventricular systolic function is normal

Atria: left atrium is mildly dilated; right atrial size is normal; no doppler evidence for an atrial septal defect

Mitral valve: mitral annular calcification; no evidence of mitral valve prolapse or valve stenosis; mild mitral regurgitation

Tricuspid valve: not well visualized but is grossly normal

Aortic valve: sclerosis mild; no hemodynamically significant valvular aortic stenosis; no aortic regurgitation is present

Pulmonic valve: not well visualized; no pulmonic valvular stenosis; mild pulmonic valvular insufficiency

Pericardium/pleural: no pericardial effusion

QUESTIONS

1. Which of the following is the main cause leading to WL's hospitalization?
   A. Heart failure exacerbation
   B. Unsafe home environment
   C. Failure to manage uncontrolled chronic disease states
   D. Overmedication

2. WL's attending physician asks you to review WL's medications given her polypharmacy. After reviewing, all of the following are issues that exists with her medication profile EXCEPT:
   A. Using medication with no indication
   B. Using medication with inappropriate dose
   C. Missing medications with mortality benefit based on past medical history
   D. Using inappropriate medication for chronic condition

3. Which of the following types of medication(s) can increase fall risk in elderly patients?
   A. Blood pressure medications
   B. Anticholinergic agents
   C. CNS depressants
   D. Antidiabetic medications
   E. Choices A, B, and C only
   F. All of the above

4. Upon reviewing WL's chart, which of the following medications should be stopped?
   A. Metformin
   B. Empagliflozin
   C. Trazodone
   D. Furosemide

5. WL presents with hypotension, which is another possible cause of falls. Which of her blood pressure medications should be the first to be discontinued?
   A. Sacubitril/valsartan
   B. Carvedilol
   C. Furosemide
   D. Clonidine

6. Which of WL's medications are on the Beers list?
   A. Clonidine
   B. Gabapentin
   C. Alprazolam
   D. Diphenhydramine
   E. Hydrocodone/acetaminophen
   F. All of the above

7. Which of the following statements is correct regarding WL's pain management?
   A. Hydrocodone/acetaminophen should be discontinued, as nonsteroidal anti-inflammatory drugs (NSAIDs) such as ketorolac or ibuprofen are the best therapy for WL.
   B. Hydrocodone/acetaminophen is the most appropriate regimen and should be continued.
   C. Hydrocodone/acetaminophen should be discontinued, as tricyclic antidepressants (TCAs) such as amitriptyline are considered first-line therapy.
   D. Hydrocodone/acetaminophen should be discontinued, as nonpharmacological methods such as exercise and multidisciplinary rehabilitation are considered first-line therapy.

8. Upon returning to the clinic for 6-month follow-up, WL's kidney function further declined (eGFR 25 mL/minute/1.73m², Scr 1.8 mg/dL). Which of the following medications does not need to be renally dosed or discontinued based on renal function?
   A. Carvedilol 25 mg PO bid
   B. Spironolactone 50 mg PO daily
   C. Metformin 1 g PO bid
   D. Empagliflozin 25 mg PO daily

REFERENCES

1. Neurontin [package insert]. New York, NY: Pfizer Inc; October 2017.
2. Baldwin D, Anderson I, Nutt D, et al. Evidence-based pharmacological treatment of anxiety disorders, posttraumatic stress disorder and obsessive-compulsive disorder: a revision of the 2005 guidelines from the British Association for Psychopharmacology. *J Psychopharmacol.* 2014;28:403-439.
3. Katzman M, Bleau P, Blier P, et al. Canadian clinical practice guidelines for the management of anxiety, posttraumatic stress and obsessive-compulsive disorders. *BMC Psychiatry.* 2014;14(suppl 1):S1-S83.
4. Fick DM, Semla TP, Steinman M, et al. American Geriatrics Society 2019 Updated AGS Beers Criteria® for Potentially Inappropriate Medication Use in Older Adults. *J Am Geriatr Soc.* 2019;67(4):674-694.
5. Yancy CW, Jessup M, Bozkurt B, et al. 2017 ACC/AHA/HFSA focused update of the 2013 ACCF/AHA guideline for the management of heart failure: a report of the American College of Cardiology/American Heart Association Task Force on Clinical Practice Guidelines and the Heart Failure Society of America. *J Am Coll Cardiol.* 2017:[Epub ahead of print].
6. National Institute for Health and Care Excellence. Low back pain and sciatica in over 16s: assessment and management. NICE Guideline 59. November 2016.
7. Toward Optimized Practice. *Guideline for Evidence-Informed Primary Care Management of Low Back Pain.* 3rd ed. December 2015.
8. Qaseem A, Wilt TJ, McLean RM, Forciea MA. Noninvasive treatments for acute, subacute, and chronic low back pain: a clinical practice guideline from the American College of Physicians. *Ann Intern Med.* 2017;166:514-530.
9. Chou R, Deyo R, Friedly J, et al. Nonpharmacologic therapies for low back pain: a systematic review for an American College of Physicians clinical practice guideline. *Ann Intern Med.* 2017;166:493-505.
10. Yancy CW, Jessup M, Bozkurt B, et al. 2017 ACC/AHA/HFSA focused update of the 2013 ACCF/AHA guideline for the management of heart failure: a report of the American College of Cardiology/American Heart Association Task Force on Clinical Practice Guidelines and the Heart Failure Society of America. *Circulation.* 2017;136(6):e137-e161.
11. Jardiance [package insert]. Ridgefield, CT: Boehringer Ingelheim Pharmaceuticals, Inc; 2020.
12. Glucophage [package insert]. Princeton, NJ: Bristol-Myers Squibb Company; 2018.

Patients Experiencing Homelessness

Phung C. On   Nikhil A. Sangave

PATIENT PRESENTATION

Medical Respite Care Admission Note

Chief Complaint

Cough, severe weakness, shortness of breath

History of Present Illness

SS is a 41-year-old male with a past medical history significant for polysubstance use and hepatitis C virus (HCV) who was admitted to our medical respite facility from a local hospital. SS was hospitalized for 3 days for management of right-sided pneumonia and polysubstance use. On admission to the medical respite, SS reports productive cough is mild with white/yellow phlegm. He denies fever, chills, and shortness of breath. He continues to have overall weakness, but it is improving. SS will remain in the medical respite for continued management of these issues.

Past Medical History

Depression
Generalized anxiety disorder
HCV (untreated)
Polysubstance use disorder (opioid, benzodiazepine, cocaine, heroin, alcohol)

Surgical History

N/A

Family History

Father: estranged; history of alcohol abuse
Mother: deceased from suicide

Social History

Smoking: current every-day smoker (0.25 packs/day).
Smokeless tobacco: denies.
Alcohol: ¼ gallon vodka/day.
Drugs: heroin (last use 1 year ago—sniffed), cocaine and methamphetamine (last used 1 month ago).
Overdose history: × 3 (2 in rapid succession when living in North Carolina, with most recent overdose ~10 months ago in Boston).
Current housing: homeless and stays between two shelters.
Family life: chaotic; father verbally abusive to him and his mother.
Abuse history: emotional, witness to domestic violence and verbal abuse.

Immunization

Pneumococcal (1 of 1, PPSV23) 10 years ago
Hepatitis B vaccine (2 of 3, Risk 3-dose series) 6 months ago

Insurance

Medicaid

Allergies

Erythromycin (hives)
Penicillin (hives)

Current Medications

Bisacodyl 10 mg suppository, 1 suppository rectally once daily as needed constipation
Bupropion XL 150 mg, 3 tablets by mouth once daily
Cefpodoxime 200 mg, 1 tablet by mouth twice daily × 2 days
Diazepam 10 mg, 1 tablet by mouth three times a day × 1 day, then 0.5 tablets three times a day × 1 day, then 0.5 tablets every 12 × 1 day, then 0.5 tablets by mouth once daily × 1 day
Docusate 100 mg, 1 capsule by mouth twice daily
Folic acid 1 mg, 1 tablet by mouth once daily

Methadone 10 mg/mL, 6.5 mL by mouth once daily
Multivitamin, 1 tablet by mouth once daily
Nicotine 14 mg/24 h, 1 patch transdermally once daily
Polyethylene glycol 17 gm, 17 gm by mouth once daily

Physical Examination

▶ Vital Signs

Temp 98.1°F, HR 71 bpm, RR 18, BP 111/70 mmHg, SpO$_2$ 95%, Ht: 6'3", Wt: 82.1 kg

▶ General

Thin-appearing, anxious male.

▶ HEENT

NC/AT.

▶ Pulmonary/Chest

Lungs cleared bilaterally, normal RR and unlabored.

▶ Cardiovascular

RRR, no m/g/r.

▶ Abdominal

Soft, nontender, nondistended, normal BS.

▶ Musculoskeletal

Normal range of motion.

▶ Neurologic

A&O × 3.

▶ Extremities

Hyperpigmented areas of prior injection to bilateral hands. No erythema or induration. No open areas.

Laboratory Findings

HAV	Reactive
HEP B S AG	Nonreactive
HEP B S AB	<5
HEP B virus core AB	Reactive
HEP C quant	1,590,000
HEP C quant log	6.20
HCV genotype	1a
HIV screen	Nonreactive

Other Results

FIB-4: F0-F1 fibrosis
PHQ-9: 11 (5 months ago)
GAD-7: 12 (5 months ago)

Hospital Discharge Summary

- Complete antibiotic treatment for pneumonia outpatient
- Continue to titrate methadone to achieve a therapeutic response
  - The patient was intermittently engaged with the methadone clinic (last dose 2 months ago at 45 mg); patient reports therapeutic dose was 70–80 mg in the past
  - During the hospital stay, methadone dose was restarted at 45 mg and titrated to 65 mg on the day of discharge
  - Patient reports using cocaine and methamphetamine up until about 1 month ago; he is feeling better now that he is off those
- Complete benzodiazepine taper
  - Patient-reported ¼ gallon vodka and 3–4 mg clonazepam use daily before hospital admission to help cope with anxiety
  - Patient presented with mild withdrawal symptoms (headache, occasional nausea, anxiety) at the hospital
  - Patient was tolerating diazepam fairly well while inpatient at the hospital but continues with headache and occasional nausea and anxiety
- HCV-untreated; patient expressed interest in starting treatment
- Behavioral health
  - Patient had seen a psychiatrist in the past but was lost to follow-up
  - Outpatient or medical respite team will need to refer the patient to behavioral health to re-establish care
- **Discharge Medications**
- Newly started
  - Cefpodoxime 200 mg, 1 tablet by mouth two times a day × 2 days
  - Diazepam 10 mg, 1 tablet by mouth three times a day × 1 day, then 0.5 tablet three times a day × 1 day, then 0.5 tablet every 12 hours × 1 day, then 0.5 tablet by mouth daily × 1 day
  - Folic acid 1 mg, 1 tablet by mouth daily
  - MVI, 1 tablet by mouth daily
  - Nicotine 14 mg/24 h, 1 patch transdermally daily
- Changed
  - Methadone 10 mg/mL, 6.5 mL by mouth daily
- Continued
  - Bisacodyl 10 mg suppository, 1 suppository rectally once daily as needed constipation
  - Bupropion XL 150 mg, 3 tablets by mouth once daily
  - Docusate 100 mg, 1 capsule by mouth twice daily
  - Naloxone 4 mg/actuation nasal spray, spray 0.1 mL into one nostril. Repeat with the second device

into the other nostril after 3 min if no or minimal response
- Polyethylene glycol 17 gm, 17 gm by mouth once daily
- Discontinued
  - Acetaminophen
  - Oxycodone

Laboratory Findings

Na = 136 mEq/L	Hgb = 12.3 g/dL	Ca = 8.2 mg/dL
K = 4.3 mEq/L	Hct = 38.5%	Albumin = 2.9 g/dL
Cl = 104 mEq/L	Plt = 404 × 10³/uL	AST = 16 IU/L
CO₂ = 24 mEq/L	WBC = 6.3 × 10³/uL	ALT = 15 IU/L
BUN = 9 mg/dL	MCV = 89 fL	T Bili = 0.3 mg/dL
SCr = 0.62 mg/dL		Alk Phos = 53 IU/L
Glu = 90 mg/dL		

Imaging

▸ **Electrocardiogram 12 lead**
- Ventricular rate 46 bpm
- Atrial rate 46 bpm
- P-R Interval 158 ms
- QRS Duration 106 ms
- QT Interval 518 ms
- QTC 453 ms

▸ **Chest X-Ray**

Bibasilar hazy retrocardiac opacities, R>L suspicious for multifocal PNA

Results Pending at Hospital Discharge

Fentanyl and norfentanyl, urine
Blood culture #1
Blood culture #2
Sputum culture

QUESTIONS

1. Which of the following most appropriately describes the features of medical respite care?
   A. Medical respite care programs are located in various settings, including nursing homes
   B. Medical respite care provides short-term medical and recuperative services for people experiencing homelessness who are not sick enough to be in a hospital but are too sick to be on the streets/shelters
   C. Medical respite care prevents unnecessary hospitalizations and reduces hospital readmissions
   D. All of the above

2. Which of the following factors may contribute to homelessness?
   A. Domestic violence
   B. Mental illness
   C. Poor health
   D. All of the above

3. If SS was discharged to the street after hospitalization instead of being admitted to the medical respite, what medication-related problem(s) might occur with his antibiotic therapy?
   A. SS completed the minimum duration of antibiotic therapy needed to treat pneumonia while in the hospital, so we do not expect to have any problems with his antibiotic therapy when he is discharged from the hospital
   B. SS may not complete antibiotic therapy if he goes back to abusing drugs or alcohol
   C. SS may not pick up the last four doses at an outpatient pharmacy in a timely manner, resulting in a lapse of antibiotic therapy
   D. Both B and C

4. SS is now ready for discharge from the medical respite. Since he will be going back to the streets/shelters, SS is at high risk for nonadherence to his medications. What medication adherence concerns do you have?
   A. SS may be lost to follow-up care, so his prescriptions for maintenance medications might not be refilled
   B. SS may not be able to afford his medications because he does not have insurance
   C. SS's medications may be compromised due to the weather
   D. Both A and C

5. Two weeks after discharge, SS attended his post-discharge follow-up appointment with his PCP. At this visit, SS noted that he wanted to start HCV treatment. Prior to starting HCV treatment, the PCP wanted to address SS's alcohol/benzodiazepine dependence. Which of the following options would be appropriate for managing SS's alcohol/benzodiazepine dependence?
   A. Start sertraline 50 mg once daily for anxiety
   B. Start naltrexone 50 mg once daily for alcohol use disorder
   C. Both A and B
   D. None of the above

6. Now that SS's polysubstance abuse has been managed, his PCP referred him to the HCV team to start HCV treatment. Which of the following medication and duration of therapy would be most appropriate for SS at this time?
   A. Ledipasvir-sofosbuvir (Harvoni) × 8 weeks
   B. Ledipasvir-sofosbuvir (Harvoni) × 12 weeks
   C. Elbasvir-grazoprevir (Zepatier) × 8 weeks
   D. Sofosbuvir-velpatasvir (Epclusa) × 8 weeks

7. The HCV team decides to place SS on ledipasvir-sofosbuvir (Harvoni) for HCV genotype 1a. Two weeks after his HCV clinic visit, SS reports to his PCP office for routine labs.

During his PCP visit, SS complains of acid reflux symptoms that have been consistent over the past week. His PCP started SS on omeprazole 20 mg daily. The prescription was sent to the pharmacy. As a verifying pharmacist, what intervention did you have to make?

A. No intervention necessary
B. Counsel SS to separate the dose of Harvoni and omeprazole by 4 hours
C. Recommend PCP to use an alternative agent such as ranitidine for acid reflux
D. Recommend PCP to switch SS's hepatitis C therapy to interferon and ribavirin

8. Patients experiencing homelessness often lose their medications or have their medications stolen. HCV treatment is expensive, so it is not easy to replace lost or stolen medications. Additionally, nonadherence to HCV treatment can be detrimental. Which of the following options can improve SS's compliance with HCV treatment and ease the cost of replacing lost medications?

A. Prescribe a short-term supply (e.g., 7 days) at a time
B. Store medications in the clinic, if feasible, and the patient would come to the clinic daily for medication
C. Prescribe enough medication supply until next lab appointment
D. All of the above

9. SS returns to the HCV clinic after 3 weeks for an adherence check-in of his HCV medications. SS attests to full adherence, which is confirmed by counting his pill bottle. SS comes back again in 3 weeks only to admit that he had missed several days of therapy. SS has since resumed his medication, but after routine labs, the viral load has increased to 3,290,000. What is the BEST intervention for the management of his HCV at this time?

A. Counsel SS on adherence and resume ledipasvir-sofosbuvir (Harvoni) for remaining duration of therapy
B. Initiate new regimen of sofosbuvir-velpatasvir-voxilaprevir (Vosevi) for 8 weeks
C. Initiate new regimen of sofosbuvir-velpatasvir-voxilaprevir (Vosevi) for 12 weeks
D. Initiate new regimen of glecaprevir/pibrentasvir (Mavyret) for 12 weeks

REFERENCES

1. National Health Care for the Homeless Council. Medical Respite Care. Available at https://nhchc.org/clinical-practice/medical-respite-care/. Nashville, TN. 2020.

2. Buchanan D, Doblin B, Sai T, Garcia P. The effects of respite care for homeless patients: a cohort study. *Am J Pub Health.* 2006;96(7):1278-1281.

3. National Health Care for the Homeless Council. Frequently Asked Questions. Available at https://nhchc.org/understanding-homelessness/faq/. Nashville, TN. 2020.

4. National Coalition for the Homeless. Homelessness in America. Available at https://nationalhomeless.org/about-homelessness/. Washington, DC. 2019.

5. AASLD-IDSA HCV Guidance Panel. Hepatitis C Guidance 2018 Update: AASLD-IDSA recommendations for testing, managing, and treating hepatitis C virus infection. *Clin Infect Dis.* 2018;67(10):1477-1492.

21 Multimodal Pain Management Strategies

Justin P. Reinert   Don Branam
Laressa Bethishou

PATIENT PRESENTATION

Chief Complaint

Motorcycle accident

History of Present Illness

US is a 41-year-old Caucasian male who presented to the emergency department (ED) 24 hours ago via EMS after suffering a motorcycle accident. According to bystanders, US hit a patch of loose gravel and was ejected from the motorcycle, landing on the pavement approximately 10 feet away. Upon presentation to the ED, US was found to have a Glasgow Coma Score (GCS) = 8 and a negative focused assessment with sonography in trauma (FAST) exam. Following a trip to the operating room for an open reduction, internal fixation (ORIF) of the left knee, US was transferred to the intensive care unit (ICU), intubated and sedated.

Past Medical History

Hypertension, hyperlipidemia

Surgical History

ORIF of left knee 12 hours ago

Family History

Unknown at present time

Social History

Unknown at present time.

Immunization History

Annual influenza vaccination, otherwise unknown at present time

Allergies

No known drug allergies

Home Medications

- HCTZ 25 mg PO daily
- Amlodipine 10 mg PO daily
- Atorvastatin 40 mg PO qHS

Current Medications

- Propofol continuous infusion, currently at 150 mcg/kg/min
- Hydromorphone continuous infusion, currently at 0.7 mg/h
- Hydromorphone 0.2 mg IV bolus PRN breakthrough pain—no doses received
- Cefazolin 1 gr IV q8h × 6 doses
- Gentamicin 5 mg/kg as a single dose—received in ED
- Heparin 5000 SQ q8h
- Lorazepam 1 mg IV q2h PRN agitation—no doses received
- Low level sliding scale insulin protocol—no doses received
- Electrolyte replacement protocol—no doses received
- Famotidine 20 mg PO bid

Physical Examination

▶ Vital Signs

Tmax since admission 99.5°F, BP 108/92 mmHg, HR 86 bpm; RR 18 breaths/min; Ht: 180 cm, Wt: 112 kg

▶ General

Intubated and sedated male patient.

▶ **HEENT**

PERRLA; otherwise deferred.

▶ **Pulmonary**

PRCV ventilation setting.

▶ **Cardiovascular**

NSR.

▶ **Abdomen**

Soft, nondistended, hypoactive bowel sounds.

▶ **Genitourinary**

Foley catheter visualized, otherwise deferred.

▶ **Neurologic**

GCS = 8 on admission, no changes appreciated. RASS = +1, CPOT = 2, CAM-ICU = negative.

▶ **Extremities**

Significant abrasions appreciated on all four extremities; fresh incision, without purulence or erythema, visualized under dressing on left knee.

Laboratory Findings

Na = 141 mEq/L	RBC = 2.5 × 10^3/mm³	Ca = 9.4 mg/dL
K = 4.8 mEq/L	WBC = 9.2 10^3/mm³	Mg = 2.4 mg/dL
Cl = 101 mEq/L	HCT = 34%	Phos = 3.5 mg/dL
CO_2 = 24 mEq/L	Plt = 116 × 10^3/mm³	Hbg = 12.2 g/dL
SCr = 2.05 mg/dL		AST = 342 IU/L
BUN = 42 mg/dL		ALT = 274 IU/L
Glucose = 138 mg/dL		

QUESTIONS

1. What is the most reliable source for collecting information on this patient's prior to admission medication list?
   A. Interviewing the patient
   B. Calling his preferred pharmacy
   C. Accessing health information exchange (HIE) from the electronic health record (EHR)
   D. Contacting his primary care physician

2. What screening tool or algorithm is used to determine if a patient is adequately sedated while mechanically ventilated?
   A. Critical Care Pain Observation Tool (CPOT)
   B. Confusion Assessment Method for the Intensive Care Unit (CAM-ICU)
   C. Richmond Agitation and Sedation Scale (RASS)
   D. CHA_2DS_2-VASc

3. US's RASS score has increased to +3 for the past 3 hours, and he is currently starting to pull at his tubes and IV lines. Which strategy is the best to help manage US's agitation?
   A. Increase propofol to 200 mcg/kg/min
   B. Increase hydromorphone to 1 mg/h
   C. Administer lorazepam 1 mg IV
   D. Initiate morphine 2 mg IV as a one-time bolus

4. A hospital policy has been approved that allows for the IV-to-PO conversion of many medications, including opioid analgesics, when considered clinically appropriate by the attending physician. You have just been consulted to make such a conversion for US. To account for incomplete cross-tolerance, hospital guidelines mandate a 25% reduction in total daily dosage with 10% of the total daily dosage reserved for breakthrough pain. Using this information, select the closest equianalgesic option.
   A. 100 mg oxycodone PO q6h and 15 mg oxycodone PO q6h PRN breakthrough pain
   B. 30 mg oxycodone PO q6h and 5 mg oxycodone PO q4h PRN breakthrough pain
   C. 75 mg oxycodone PO q6h and 20 mg oxycodone PO q6h PRN breakthrough pain
   D. 25 mg oxycodone PO q6h and 50 mg oxycodone PO q6h PRN breakthrough pain

5. During one of US's spontaneous breathing and awakening trials, he informs the medical team that he has a history of substance and has previously spent time in rehabilitation for opioid abuse. He requests that he does not receive any additional opioids. Unfortunately, his breathing becomes labored and he is sedated, with his ventilator settings restored. Using this information, which describes the best alternative regimens for US?
   A. Initiate a ketamine infusion at 1 mcg/kg/min; wean off hydromorphone infusion and maintain propofol infusion and titrate to RASS of −1 to +1
   B. Initiate dexmedetomidine infusion at 0.2 mcg/kg/h; wean off hydromorphone infusion and wean off propofol infusion
   C. Wean off hydromorphone infusion and initiate a midazolam infusion at 1 mg/h; maintain propofol infusion and titrate to RASS of −1 to +1
   D. Initiate a pentobarbital infusion at 1 mg/kg/h; wean off hydromorphone infusion and wean off propofol infusion

6. It has been 5 days since US came to the ICU. He was successfully extubated yesterday morning and he is no longer receiving his continuous infusion medications; however, he remains agitated to the point that his breathing becomes labored. As such, US has been receiving dexmedetomidine at 0.5 mcg/kg/h for the past 24 hours, but is now ready to transfer to the floor, where dexmedetomidine is prohibited by hospital policy. Based on US's situation, which of the following regimens provides the best options for US's analgesic and sedative needs?
   A. Lidocaine patches applied 12 hours on, 12 hours off + methocarbamol 500 mg PO q6h PRN
   B. Ibuprofen 600 mg PO q8h + clonidine 0.1 mg PO tid + tizanidine 4 mg PO tid + pregabalin 75 mg PO daily

C. Oxycodone 5 mg PO q4-6h PRN + acetaminophen 1000 mg PO q6h + diazepam 10 mg PO daily

D. Acetaminophen 500 mg PO q6h + clonidine 0.1 mg PO tid + cyclobenzaprine 5 mg PO tid + gabapentin 200 mg PO tid

7. US has been on the medical/surgical floor for 24 hours. He has been out of bed briefly to a bedside chair. His nurse reports that he has not had a bowel movement in 3 days. He denies any abdominal discomfort, but his abdomen is mildly distended. He is afebrile and the rest of his vital signs are within normal limits. What is the most likely cause of US's constipation, and what is a reasonable alternative therapy for pain management?

A. Acetaminophen; change to ibuprofen 400 mg PO tid

B. Clonidine; change to tizanidine 4 mg PO tid

C. Cyclobenzaprine; change to methocarbamol 1000 mg PO tid

D. Gabapentin; change to pregabalin 25 mg PO tid

8. US' constipation is relieved with the administration of a rectal enema. Two of his home medications, atorvastatin and amlodipine, are reinitiated, with amlodipine started at 2.5 mg by mouth daily. Today is now his second day on the medical/surgical floor, and his vital signs are: Temp 37.1°C, HR 62 beats/minute, BP 92/48 mmHg, RR 18 breaths/minute. Which of the following interventions should be recommended at this time?

A. Reduce acetaminophen to 325 mg every 6 hours

B. Reduce clonidine to 0.05 mg three times daily

C. Discontinue amlodipine

D. Discontinue atorvastatin

9. On day 3 of US' stay on the medical/surgical floor, plans are underway to transfer him to a skilled nursing facility (SNF) for continued rehabilitation and care. His pain management is adequate considering his injuries, and he is calm on his current regimen. The physical therapist reports that his ambulation has improved; however, he still requires moderate assistance when getting out of bed. What changes in his pain regimen should be considered upon transfer to a SNF?

A. Decrease clonidine to 0.05 mg twice daily, continue acetaminophen, amlodipine, atorvastatin, and methocarbamol at current dosages

B. Discontinue clonidine, decrease methocarbamol to 500 mg three times daily, decrease gabapentin to 100 mg three times daily, increase amlodipine to 5 mg daily, and continue acetaminophen and atorvastatin at current dosages

C. Decrease clonidine to 0.05 mg twice daily, discontinue methocarbamol, reinitiate HCTZ at 25 mg daily, increase amlodipine to 5 mg PO daily, and continue acetaminophen, atorvastatin, and gabapentin at current dosages

D. Discontinue clonidine and methocarbamol, increase amlodipine to 5 mg PO daily, and continue acetaminophen, atorvastatin at current dosages

10. Based upon US's hospital course and any relevant past medical history, what vaccination would be best to administer to US before he is transferred to the SNF?

A. Hepatitis B vaccine series; give first dose in series now

B. Zoster vaccine

C. Tetanus and diphtheria toxoids and acellular pertussis vaccine (Tdap) "booster" vaccination

D. Human papillomavirus vaccination

REFERENCES

1. Canadian Patient Safety Institute: Best Possible Medication History. Available at https://www.patientsafetyinstitute.ca/en/Topic/Pages/Best-Possible-Medication-History.aspx. 2020.

2. Sessler CN, Grap MJ, Ramsay MA. Evaluating and monitoring analgesia and sedation in the intensive care unit. *Crit Care.* 2008;12(suppl 3):S2.

3. Devlin JW, Skrobik Y, Gélinas C, et al. Clinical practice guidelines for the prevention and management of pain, agitation/sedation, delirium, immobility, and sleep disruption in adult patients in the ICU. *Crit Care Med.* 2018;46(9):e825-e873.

4. Riggi F, Glass M. Update on the management and monitoring of deep analgesia and sedation in the intensive care unit. *AACN Adv Crit Care.* 2013; 24(2):101-107.

5. Zhu WG, Xiong QM, Hong K. Meta-analysis of CHADS2 versus CHA2DS2-VASc for predicting stroke and thromboembolism in atrial fibrillation patients independent of anticoagulation. *Tex Heart Inst J.* 2015;42(1):6-15.

6. Wiatrowski R, Norton C, Giffen D. Analgosedation: improving patient outcomes in ICU sedation and pain management. *Pain Manag Nurs.* 2016;17(3):204-217.

7. Murray A, Hagen NA. Hydromorphone. *J Pain Symptom Manage.* 2005;29(suppl 5):S57-S66.

8. Zaal IJ, Devlin JW, Hazelbag M, et al. Benzodiazepine-associated delirium in critically ill adults. *Intensive Care Med.* 2015;41(12):2130-2137.

9. Smith HS, Peppin JF. Toward a systematic approach to opioid rotation. *J Pain Res.* 2014;7:589-608.

10. Natusch D. Equianalgesic doses of opioids - their use in clinical practice. *Br J Pain.* 2012;6(1):43-46.

11. Dumas EO, Pollack GM. Opioid tolerance development: a pharmacokinetic/pharmacodynamic perspective. *AAPS J.* 2008;10(4):537-551.

12. Reade MC, Finfer S. Sedation and delirium in the intensive care unit. *N Engl J Med.* 2014;370(5):444-454.

13. Patel SB, Kress JP. Sedation and analgesia in the mechanically ventilated patient. *Am J Respir Crit Care Med.* 2012;185(5):486-497.

14. Ingalls NK, Horton ZA, Bettendorf M, et al. Randomized, double-blind, placebo-controlled trial using lidocaine patch 5% in traumatic rib fractures. *J Am Coll Surg.* 2010;210(2):205-209.

15. Zhao-Fleming H, Hand A, Zhang K, et al. Effect of non-steroidal anti-inflammatory drugs on post-surgical

complications against the backdrop of the opioid crisis. *Burns Trauma.* 2018;6:25.

16. Publow SW, Branam DL. Hypotension and bradycardia associated with concomitant tizanidine and lisinopril therapy. *Am J Health Syst Pharm.* 2010;67(19): 1606-1610.

17. Terry K, Blum R, Szumita P. Evaluating the transition from dexmedetomidine to clonidine for agitation management in the intensive care unit. *SAGE Open Med.* 2015;3:2050312115621767.

18. Gagnon DJ, Riker RR, Glisic EK, et al. Transition from dexmedetomidine to enteral clonidine for ICU sedation: an observational pilot study. *Pharmacotherapy.* 2015;35(3):251-259.

19. Beebe F, Barkin R, Barkin S. A clinical and pharmacologic review of skeletal muscle relaxants for musculoskeletal conditions. *Am J Therapeut.* 2005;12:151-171.

20. Ozawa Y, Hayashi K, Kobori H. New generation calcium channel blockers in hypertensive treatment. *Curr Hypertens Rev.* 2006;2(2):103-111.

21. MacDougall AI, Addis GJ, Mackay N, et al. Treatment of hypertension with clonidine. *BMJ.* 1970;3(5720): 440–442.

22. Cauley JA, Cummings SR, Seeley DG, et al. Effects of thiazide diuretic therapy on bone mass, fractures, and falls. The study of the Osteoporotic Fractures Research Group. *Ann Intern Med.* 1993;118(9):666-673.

23. Schillie S, Harris A, Gelles-Link R, et al. Recommendations of the Advisory Committee on Immunization Practices for use of a hepatitis B vaccine with a novel adjuvant. *MMWR.* 2017:67(15):455-488.

24. Dooling KL, Guo A, Patel M, et al. Recommendations of the Advisory Committee on Immunization Practices for use of herpes zoster vaccines. *MMWR.* 2018:67(3):103-108.

25. Meites E, Szilagyi PG, Chesson HW, et al. Human papillomavirus vaccination for adults: updated recommendations of the Advisory Committee on Immunization Practices. *MMWR.* 2019;68(32):698-702.

26. Havers FP, Moro PD, Hunter P, et al. Use of tetanus toxoid, reduced diphtheria toxoid, and acellular pertussis vaccines: updated recommendations of the Advisory Committee on Immunization Practices. *MMWR.* 2020;69(3):77-83.

27. Yorkgitis BK, Timoney G, Salim A, et al. Pertussis vaccination in adult trauma patients: are we missing an opportunity? *Surgery.* 2015;158(3):602-607.

22 Complexities of Managing Psychiatric Pharmacotherapy

Brittany L. Parmentier   Jessica Wooster

PATIENT PRESENTATION

Chief Complaint

"They are trying to poison me."

History of Present Illness

LM is a 38-year-old male who is brought to the emergency department by a staff member of his group home. The patient complains that staff at his group home are trying to poison him. He states that he has stopped eating and taking his medications because of this. He states that he hears voices that tell him not to eat because the staff are "out to get me." Group home staff report that the patient has not been eating his meals for 3 days, even with significant prompting.

Past Psychiatric History

Diagnosed with schizophrenia at age 22. Patient has been hospitalized for psychiatric symptoms four times in his life. Patient was started on clozapine 9 months ago and was doing well in his group home according to staff. Past medication trials of olanzapine, paliperidone, risperidone, and ziprasidone were unsuccessful.

Past Medical/Surgical History

Obesity
Hyperlipidemia
Hypertension

Family History

Uncle from his mother's side has schizophrenia
Mother has anxiety disorder

Social History

Single and unemployed.
Lives in a group home.

Immunization

Up to date

Insurance

State Medicaid; medication coverage is not a problem

Allergies

No known drug allergies

Home Medications

- Clozapine 150 mg PO bid
- Atorvastatin 20 mg PO at bedtime
- Lisinopril 20 mg PO daily
- Hydroxyzine pamoate 50 mg every 6 hours PRN anxiety

Physical Examination

▷ *General*

Overweight, disheveled male appearing stated age.

Mental Status Examination

▷ *Appearance/Behavior/Speech*

Grooming and hygiene were poor. Patient was observed attending to internal stimuli. Speech was normal rate and quiet volume at times. No psychomotor abnormalities appreciated.

▷ *Mood/Affect*

Patient describes his mood as "fine." His affect was flat, constricted, non-labile, but congruent with stated mood.

▷ *Sensorium*

Awake and alert, appears grossly oriented, but not formally tested.

▶ **Intellectual functioning**

Not formally tested. Average based upon vocabulary and general fund of knowledge.

▶ **Attention/Concentration**

Unable to maintain attention and concentration during the interview.

▶ **Memory**

Not formally tested, appears intact based on ability to recall and discuss recent events.

▶ **Thought Process/Content**

Thoughts are disorganized and illogical. Auditory hallucinations of voices telling him not to eat. He reports persecutory delusions. He does not endorse suicidal ideations.

▶ **Judgment/Insight**

Poor/Poor.

▶ **Vital Signs**

Temp 98.5°F, P 65 beats per minute, RR 18 breaths per minute, BP 123/89 mmHg, pO_2 99%, Ht: 5'9", Wt: 109.1 kg

Laboratory Values

WBC = $6.44 \times 10^3/\mu L$	
Hgb = 15.3 g/dL	
Hct = 48.5%	
Plt = $250 \times 10^3/\mu L$	
RBC = $4.62 \times 10^6/\mu L$	
Neut = 65%	
Lymph = 26.3%	
Mono = 5.8%	
Eos = 0.8%	
Baso = 0.6	

Urine Drug Screen

Negative

Assessment

Schizophrenia, multiple episodes, currently in acute episode.

Plan

Admit to acute inpatient psychiatric unit for stabilization; restart all of patient's home medications.

QUESTIONS

1. As the inpatient clinical pharmacist, you want to determine when the patient last took a dose of clozapine. Which of the following resources would be best to determine this information based on the patient?
   A. Ask the patient
   B. Call the patient's parents and ask
   C. Call the pharmacy that dispenses the clozapine
   D. Obtain the medication administration records from the group home

2. You determine that LM last took a dose of his clozapine 3 days prior to admission. What dose of clozapine would you recommend restarting on admission for LM?
   A. 12.5 mg twice daily
   B. 50 mg twice daily
   C. 150 mg twice daily
   D. 200 mg twice daily

3. Clozapine should be restarted at the starting dose after how many days without taking the medication?
   A. 2 days
   B. 5 days
   C. 10 days
   D. 30 days

4. What side effect could occur if LM is restarted immediately on his home dose of clozapine 150 mg twice daily instead of the initial recommended dose?
   A. Severe neutropenia
   B. Orthostasis
   C. Hepatotoxicity
   D. Hypoglycemia

5. The patient has been restarted on an appropriate dose of clozapine, but the nurse reports to the psychiatrist and pharmacist that they are worried the patient is not swallowing his medications, and instead is holding them in his mouth and spitting them in the toilet later. Which of the following changes could be made to potentially improve the patient's medication adherence?
   A. Continue to increase the clozapine dose every day
   B. Change the clozapine tablets to paliperidone tablets
   C. Continue the starting dose of clozapine tablets until you can ensure the patient is adherent
   D. Change the clozapine tablets to orally disintegrating tablets

6. Before being admitted to the hospital, the patient had his absolute neutrophil count (ANC) labs drawn for the Clozapine Risk Evaluation and Mitigation Strategy (REMS) program every 2 weeks. How frequently should the ANC lab monitoring be performed once he restarts clozapine?
   A. Three times weekly
   B. Weekly
   C. Every 2 weeks
   D. Monthly

7. The patient is restarted on his clozapine appropriately. During the inpatient admission, his dose was increased to clozapine 200 mg PO bid. The team is now preparing for discharge, but the patient will be discharging to a different

group home than the one he lived in prior to admission. The new group home will manage the medications and give LM his medications at the appropriate time. Which of the following steps can the inpatient pharmacist take to best ensure that patient hand-off to his new group home is effective?

A. Verify that the community pharmacy that fills medications for the new group home is certified in the Clozapine REMS program

B. Verify that the new group home is certified in the Clozapine REMS program to administer clozapine

C. Call the patient's family and ask them to transfer the old clozapine prescription to the new community pharmacy

D. Ask the inpatient psychiatrist to print a paper copy of the clozapine prescription for the patient to take to his new pharmacy

8. The inpatient psychiatrist is going to send a prescription for clozapine to the new community pharmacy. How many days' supply of the clozapine can the community pharmacy dispense for LM?

A. 7 days

B. 14 days

C. 30 days

D. As many days as the patient's insurance allows

9. Which of the following education points is most important to provide to LM prior to discharge to the group home?

A. LM needs to have more frequent lab monitoring because the dose of clozapine was increased

B. LM will need to bring his lab results with him to the pharmacy to get his clozapine

C. LM should continue to take the clozapine, even if he feels better

D. LM is at a high risk for neutropenia because of the dose of clozapine

10. LM has a new psychiatrist at his new group home. When the psychiatrist sends his next clozapine prescription to the pharmacy, the pharmacist learns that the new prescriber is not certified in the Clozapine REMS program. What step can the pharmacist take to ensure LM does not have a treatment interruption?

A. Dispense the clozapine without any further documentation

B. Call LM's new psychiatrist and tell her she needs to become certified in the Clozapine REMS program before clozapine can be dispensed

C. Call LM's recent inpatient psychiatrist and ask him to send another prescription for clozapine

D. Provide a "Dispense Rationale" in the Clozapine REMS program and dispense the clozapine

REFERENCES

1. Clozaril® [full prescribing information]. Rosemont, PA: HLS Therapeutics (USA), Inc.; March 2020.

2. Clozapine and the Risk of Neutropenia: A Guide for Healthcare Providers. Clozapine REMS. Available at https://www.clozapinerems.com/CpmgClozapineUI/rems/pdf/resources/Clozapine_REMS_A_Guide_for_Healthcare_Providers.pdf. Published February 2019. Accessed June 4, 2020.

3. Keepers GA, Fochtmann LJ, Anzia JM, et al. The American Psychiatric Association practice guideline for the treatment of patients with schizophrenia. American Psychiatric Association. Available at https://www.psychiatry.org/psychiatrists/practice/clinical-practice-guidelines. Published December 2019. Accessed June 4, 2020.

4. PDA Fact Sheet for Outpatient Pharmacies. Clozapine REMS. Available at https://www.clozapinerems.com/CpmgClozapineUI/rems/pdf/resources/Clozapine_REMS_PDA_Fact_Sheet.pdf. Published February 2019. Accessed June 4, 2020.

Answers with Rationales

CASE 1

1. **Correct answer: A**

   Rationale: At each care transition, patients will have a different set of needs that the pharmacist must address. Upon admission to the ED, this includes collection of a best possible medication history and admission medication reconciliation. The BPMH should include a comprehensive list of all medications the patient is taking, including over-the-counter medications and supplements. It should also include an assessment of adherence to inquire how the patient is actually taking their medications, and identify if, and why, the patient may be taking medications differently than prescribed. A patient interview is preferred, with verification from a second source, as the patient can provide the most comprehensive and up-to-date information as well as identify any adherence issues. In this case, the patient lives alone and seems to be managing her own health. There is no indication that the patient is an unreliable historian, such as confusion or involvement of a caregiver, although it would be important to collect this information and identify if any other caregivers or co-learners should be involved in decision-making and education. There is also no indication that her daughter is directly involved with her care. Pharmacy records and medical records from a physician are also excellent resources to verify patient medication lists but may not provide a comprehensive picture.

2. **Correct answer: D**

   Rationale: In order to comprehensively address the patient's needs, we must assess the information we have collected to conduct an accurate assessment of the patient's current problem. We must consider how this patient's health information impacts interventions including medication reconciliation, therapy planning and implementation, patient education, adherence barriers, and care coordination. The patient has been taking ibuprofen twice daily for back pain since her fall 2 months ago. Additionally, she has been taking Alka Seltzer, which contains 325 mg of aspirin per tablet, to ease her "stomach upset." Excessive NSAID use can cause a peptic ulcer and increased risk of gastrointestinal bleed, which is consistent with the patient's clinical presentation of tarry stools and vomiting coffee-ground emesis. While stress, weight gain, and an *H. pylori* infection can all be causes of noncardiac chest pain and peptic ulcers, there is no evidence that these were contributors for the patient. This will be significant to the assessment and plan, as we will need to treat her symptoms, optimize her medication lists to remove medications that contribute to her current symptoms, and address any other complaints that may impact her health, such as the back pain that prompted her to take NSAIDs in the first place, and even the confusion that led to her fall.

3. **Correct answer: D**

   Rationale: TOC interventions for this patient will include admission medication reconciliation, medication therapy optimization, and comprehensive discharge planning. In addition to collecting a BPMH, which will support these activities, we would like to collect any additional information that will guide us in providing care to this patient and supporting safe and effective care transitions as she moves through her hospitalization. At this care transition, we will need to initiate therapy to manage her epigastric pain and vomiting. Based on her past medical history, history of present illness, and her clinical presentation, we can select the appropriate medications but we need to know if the patient can take oral medications. Her NPO status will guide the route we select. It is always important to ensure the patient is able to access and administer medications we select, so consideration of route, along with other access barriers, is important. We also want to optimize her medication therapy regimen, so any information about health problems, medications, and potential adverse effects will be important to us. In this case, the patient reports taking an over-the-counter medication, Tylenol PM, because she has trouble sleeping. This is important for several reasons. The elderly patient is taking an over-the-counter medication with diphenhydramine, which should be avoided per Beers criteria.[4] The patient had a fall 2 months ago, and medications which can affect cognitive ability and increase fall risk, such as antihistamines, should be avoided. Additionally, the patient complains about difficulty sleeping but takes her fluoxetine with dinner. This may be contributing to her difficulty sleeping, as fluoxetine is activating and should be taken in the morning. The medication reconciliation and patient education for this patient will need to address these points.

4. **Correct answer: D**

   Rationale: The patient has noncardiac chest pain secondary to her peptic ulcer. Because she has been taking high doses of NSAIDs to manage her back pain and taking aspirin to manage the associated stomach pain, she has developed a peptic ulcer. Therefore, we must initiate treatment to treat her ulcer, manage her symptoms, and prevent recurrence. It is important to identify the treatment goals when we assess and identify appropriate therapy. In this case, that will involve ruling out an active bleed, which we can do because the patient has tarry black stools. The most appropriate treatment for noncardiac chest pain secondary to NSAID use is a PPI, which is dosed double the standard dose for management of noncardiac chest pain.[5] Options A and B doses are too low for this patient. Additionally, the patient has an NPO order and is vomiting, so oral medication would not be appropriate at this time, ruling out options A and C.

5. **Correct answer: C**

   Rationale: Noncardiac chest pain should be treated with a PPI for at least 2 months.[5] At that point, we can consider reducing the dose and reassessing appropriateness of therapy. In creating and implementing a plan for the patient, duration of therapy and required follow-up and monitoring should be taken into consideration.

6. **Correct answer: C**

   Rationale: Assessing immunization status during care transitions is an important intervention to optimize health outcomes, especially if patients are elderly or have comorbidities that make them more susceptible or vulnerable to the effects of common illnesses. The patient is over the age of 65 and has an indication for Pneumovax based on her age. Although patients over 65 may decide to get Prevnar 13, the patient is not immunocompromised and she does not have any of the medical conditions that would require her to get Prevnar 13.[6] She also has an indication for herpes zoster vaccine based on her age. Shingrix is preferred over Zostavax as it has evidence of greater efficacy.[6] Therefore, to meet her treatment goals and optimize her care, we should administer appropriate vaccines.

7. **Correct answer: C**

   Rationale: Implementing the plan requires interventions to put it into action. This includes ordering medications, educating the patient, and coordinating follow-up. Since we have identified that increased NSAID use and Alka Seltzer are contributing to her peptic ulcer, these should be discontinued. Her new PPI will treat her stomach pain, so there is no indication for Alka Seltzer. The patient mentions she was taking the NSAID for back pain secondary to a fall. She also mentions she takes her fluoxetine at night and uses Tylenol PM to help with sleep. Therefore, the actionable items include addressing these. Fluoxetine should be taken in the morning, as the medication is activating and may be the cause for her difficulty sleeping. We should discontinue the Tylenol PM, as this may have contributed to her fall, but should not start a sleep aid in its place.

8. **Correct answer: D**

   Rationale: At follow-up, healthcare providers should evaluate the safety and effectiveness of medications to ensure optimal health outcomes and progress toward achievement of treatment goals. Since we started the patient on a higher dose of PPI for management of noncardiac chest pain, we want to evaluate the efficacy but also minimize the risk of adverse outcomes. Long-term PPI use is associated with adverse events, including increased risk of pneumonia and *Clostridium difficile* infection, as well as decreased calcium absorption.[7] When appropriate, we can decrease the PPI dose, as the patient does have osteoporosis. We may want to check her calcium levels, consider calcium supplementation, and ensure the PPI is decreased in dose, or even discontinued, when appropriate. Since her symptoms were precipitated by NSAID use secondary to back pain, she may not have an indication for long-term PPI use. Additionally, we want to ensure her back pain is properly addressed at the follow-up appointment so the patient will not require NSAIDs for pain management.

CASE 2

1. **Correct answer: D**

   Rationale: Medication reconciliation should be completed at all care transitions whether within the same setting or in different settings.[1,2] While in the hospital, medication reconciliation should be completed on admission to the hospital, when the patient is transferred between services or units, and on discharge. The same process would apply if the patient was admitted and discharged from a post-acute care facility such as a skilled nursing facility. If a patient is seeing a healthcare provider in the outpatient setting, medication reconciliation should be completed at every visit.

2. **Correct answer: C**

   Rationale: When obtaining a medication list from the patient or caregiver, the interviewer should begin with open-ended questions and use layman's terms.[3] Although option D is an open-ended question, hypertension is a medical term, thus this option is incorrect. Options A and B are closed-ended questions and therefore these options are incorrect. Rephrasing option A and B to state, "What medications do you take at home for your high blood pressure?" would be more appropriate.

3. **Correct answer: D**

   Rationale: When completing a medication reconciliation, it is important to obtain the appropriate medication list(s) prior to coming up with the best possible medication list for the patient. These medication lists should include a list of medications the patient is taking. If KR is taking care of his own medications, interviewing him would be appropriate. However, KR is living at an assisted living facility and has early-onset dementia. Patients living at assisted living facilities have personnel who assist with their medication administration. Thus, interviewing KR would not be appropriate (option B). Instead, we would want to contact the assisted living facility to determine what medication the patient is taking (option A). Further, we want to use the medication list from the current clinical encounter as another source of medication list (option C).

4. **Correct answer: B**

   Rationale: An error of omission is defined as a medication that should have been administered, prescribed, or dispensed but was omitted from the orders.[3] It is unclear why amlodipine was not restarted in the hospital. Thus, option B is correct. Although lisinopril was not restarted in the hospital, you can safely assume that lisinopril was held due to elevated potassium levels (option D). Starting or restarting a medication such as acetaminophen or latanoprost in the hospital would not be an error of omission (options A and C, respectively).

5. **Correct answer: D**
   Rationale: An error of commission is defined as a medication prescribed, dispensed, or given incorrectly with no indication.[3] It is unclear why omeprazole was started in the hospital. The patient does not have an indication for omeprazole; therefore option D is correct. Atorvastatin was started in the hospital as a therapeutic substitution for rosuvastatin (option A). Patient underwent surgery, so hydrocodone/acetaminophen was ordered for postoperative pain (option B). Not restarting calcium carbonate/vitamin D is potentially an error of omission, not commission (option C). However, it is appropriate to hold calcium carbonate/vitamin D while the patient is hospitalized.

6. **Correct answer: D**
   Rationale: It is appropriate to hold capsaicin while the patient is hospitalized, as it was prescribed to help with KR's left hip pain. Since the patient is recovering from THA, he requires stronger oral pain medications, and capsaicin should not be used on any open wounds such as a surgical incision (option A). It is appropriate to start regular insulin per sliding scale, as the patient would need something to help control his blood sugar since the hospital team held metformin (option B). Metformin is often held at hospital admission in case patients are exposed to iodine contrast studies during the hospital stay, to avoid adverse effects. It is appropriate to not restart rosuvastatin, since atorvastatin was started in the hospital (option C). Atorvastatin is an appropriate therapeutic substitution for rosuvastatin, and the change was likely due to hospital formulary.

7. **Correct answer: A**
   Rationale: There is no reason to hold allopurinol during the hospital stay, so option B is incorrect. Allopurinol is used for the prevention of gout flareups by chronically lowering the uric acid levels and is not meant to treat acute gout flares; therefore options C and D are incorrect.

8. **Correct answer: D**
   Rationale: Orthopedic surgeries including THA put patients at high risk for venous thromboembolism (VTE). As a result, anticoagulation is often recommended for prevention of VTE post-operation. Substituting heparin with rivaroxaban in the outpatient setting is appropriate (option A). Options B and C are both accurate counseling points for rivaroxaban and should be discussed with the patient. Patients should also be counseled on the specific signs and symptoms of bleeding such as unusual bleeding, coughing up blood, dark tarry stool, feeling dizzy or weak, etc.[4]

9. **Correct answer: C**
   Rationale: The Omnibus Budget Reconciliation Act of 1987 (OBRA-87) set standards related to pharmacy practice for nursing facilities accepting Medicare and Medicaid funding. OBRA-87 stated that a licensed pharmacist must perform a drug regimen review (DRR) at least once per month; therefore options A, B, and D are incorrect. Any findings from the DRR must be reported to the attending physician or director of nursing.[5]

CASE 3

1. **Correct answer: D**
   Rationale: At hospital discharge, transitions of care activities include medication reconciliation, patient education, comprehensive discharge planning, care coordination, and identifying and resolving medication access barriers. While we do have a prior-to-admission medication list, our patient was confused on admission. Therefore, it would be helpful to collect additional information that may be pertinent to our discharge medication reconciliation. This includes information on adherence issues, timing of last doses including her weekly alendronate, and any additional medications including over-the-counter and supplements which may interact with her existing medications. If our patient takes additional medications, this needs to be considered when reconciling her medications. Sleep medications may be contributing to her confusion and may be inappropriate given her age. We also want to consider any barriers to proper medication use or accessing patient care. This includes impaired functional status. If our patient has difficulty getting around her house, she may need evaluation by physical therapy. This is important in both supporting access to care and in assessing fall risk. Since our patient is widowed, lives alone, and presented with complaints of confusion and difficulty managing her medications, we should consider the level of support and caregiver involvement. This may be helpful in determining who should be present when educating the patient, but it may also determine whether we should collaborate with case management or social work to identify additional resources to help the patient with follow-up and management of her medications. This can include strategies such as helping her fill her pill box, identifying medications which are unnecessary or can be de-prescribed, or connecting the patient with additional support such as home health resources. Since her daughter helps her fill her pill box, she should be included in any discussions and education about medications and caregiver support.

2. **Correct answer: C**
   Rationale: Over-the-counter (OTC) medications, including supplements, are not always reported. It is often assumed they are safe because they do not require a prescription. It is important to evaluate OTC medications for drug interactions and adverse effects. Additionally, our patient came in confused, so we should assess whether her OTC medications may be contributing to her symptoms. Lastly, the patient complains of difficulty managing her

medications. Therefore, if we can discontinue medications that are not necessary, that is valuable. These medications are not all appropriate for the patient so they should each be evaluated for appropriate indication, drug interactions, and adverse effects. While St. John's Wort does not cause confusion, there is no clear indication for it, as the patient denies depression. If the patient is taking this for mood, we can refer her to her primary care provider for evaluation and treatment. Her Excedrin has caffeine, which may be affecting sleep and requiring the patient to take sleep aids. We can clarify the indication with the patient and support her in selecting an appropriate OTC agent which will not affect sleep. Lastly, our patient is taking multiple sleep aids which contain diphenhydramine. These should both be discontinued as antihistamines are not recommended in elderly patients per the Beers Criteria. These may be contributing to her confusion and dizziness and can increase fall risk.

3. **Correct answer: A**
   Rationale: Comprehensive discharge planning should be interprofessional and collaborative, and serve to anticipate and address patient specific needs. Our patient's gait has not been assessed yet, but she complains of difficulty getting around the house. She also has increased fall risk due to her dizziness and confusion. Therefore, she would benefit from an evaluation by physical and occupational therapists to identify functional mobility and level of support needed around the house. While ensuring that coverage of medications and appropriate prescribing is important, we should extend this to all medications, not just newly prescribed ones. To prevent readmissions and ensure continuity of care, we seek to identify any adherence barriers such as cost, no refills, or incorrectly prescribed medications. If the patient is not taking prior-to-admission medications because they are out of refills or not able to afford them, this should be addressed. The patient may also benefit from coordination of home health services. While the patient and her family are valuable members of the patient care team, and should absolutely be engaged, discharge planning should support them by helping meet their care needs. Therefore, we would not ask the daughter to take ownership of finding home health services. We could instead collaborate with case management and social work to assess patient needs and set up home health services prior to discharge.

4. **Correct answer: C**
   Rationale: Discharge medication reconciliation should compare her prior to admission medication, inpatient, and discharge medication lists. Based on her treatment goals for each active problem, her changes to health status and labs, and any access or adherence barriers, the most appropriate medications should be determined. The patient was started on levofloxacin for suspected UTI in the hospital and would require 3 doses to complete her course of treatment (since she was admitted yesterday, this would mean 1 to 2 additional doses). However, her UA was

clear and her confusion resolved. Therefore, there is no indication to discharge with an antibiotic. The patient also had her amlodipine held during her hospitalization due to low blood pressure. Therefore, it would be appropriate to continue holding her amlodipine at this time given her hypotension. Lastly, the patient is on brand-name Synthroid prior to admission. While generic is used during her admission, there can be variability in brand and generic dosing for thyroid medication and they should not be used interchangeably. Therefore, her home regimen should be resumed.

5. **Correct answer: B**
   Rationale: Discharge medication education should provide a comprehensive overview of the patient's discharge medication list. While this certainly includes a thorough review of new medications, the entire medication list should be reviewed. Patients should be educated on new medications, changes to their medication list, and medications which are discontinued. For each medication, they should be provided with the name, indication, dosing, route, frequency, and any relevant education on administration, storage, adverse effects, drug interactions, and necessary follow-up and monitoring. It may be helpful to explain the purpose of the education session so the patient is aware what will be covered and can follow along. Using open-ended questions and incorporating teach-back are valuable techniques to engage the patient and assess their understanding and where there may be need for reinforcement. Education should include any family or caregivers who are helping manage medication. If the patient has language barriers, an interpreter should be included in the education as well. This may require coordinating discharge education in advance, to ensure all parties are present. In this case, there is no indication the patient speaks a second language or requires an interpreter present. If the patient does speak a second language, we can ask the patient if they would like an interpreter present and coordinate accordingly. Most hospitals will have in-person, telephone, or virtual language interpretation services available.

6. **Correct answer: D**
   Rationale: Women should limit their daily alcohol intake to one serving of alcohol per day. This patient currently drinks one to two glasses of brandy per day. Alcohol serving size should also be defined for the patient, as 1.5 oz of distilled spirits constitutes one serving. Alcohol consumption may also be contributing to the patient's confusion and therefore should be limited (answer A). The patient is currently taking several medications that may interact with one another and have specific requirements for appropriate administration times. Taking calcium and metoprolol tartrate together is not a concern (answer B). Confirm if the patient is aware of the following administration recommendations: levothyroxine should be taken first thing in the morning on an empty stomach at least 30 to 60 minutes before food. Alternatively, may consistently administer at night 3 to 4 hours after the last meal. Levothyroxine and

calcium should be separated by at least 4 hours as calcium may suppress the therapeutic effect of levothyroxine. Alendronate should be administered on an empty stomach at least 30 minutes prior to food, beverages, or medications—not with calcium (answer C). Patient should stay upright for at least 30 minutes to prevent esophageal irritation. The patient should be counseled on proper sleep hygiene as she has indicated she has problems sleeping and has taken OTC sleep aids in the past. Good sleep habits can improve mental and physical health. After establishing good sleep habits, if trouble with sleep still occurs, referral to her PCP would be warranted (answer D).

7. **Correct answer: D**
   Rationale: Amlodipine was held during admission. Her blood pressure remains low at discharge and should be monitored and followed up to assess if discontinuing amlodipine remains appropriate. The patient also presented with dizziness, which can be a sign of hypotension. It should be assessed if the patient has a blood pressure monitor at home and the patient should be educated on proper blood pressure monitoring technique (answer A). The patient was taking St. John's Wort OTC and needs to be assessed if she has a true indication for it. It would be appropriate to ask the patient if she knows what she is taking it for; whether the patient knows the indication or not, she should follow up with her PCP for assessment and to determine the appropriateness of continuing this medication (answer B). It is always important for the patient to be followed up regarding symptoms that brought her to the hospital in the first place to ensure she is not experiencing a repeat of symptoms that could lead to another hospitalization (answer C).

CASE 4

1. **Correct answer: D**
   Rationale: The back pain the patient is experiencing is not a sign or symptom of GERD. He is needing to sleep in the recliner due to his GERD symptoms at night that worsen while lying flat, thus it is the sleeping position causing the back pain. Answers A through C are all signs and symptoms of GERD.[1]

2. **Correct answer: A**
   Rationale: Alarm symptoms for GERD that should result in a patient referral to a physician include dysphagia, odynophagia (painful swallowing), recurrent bronchial symptoms, aspiration pneumonia, dysphonia, recurrent or persistent cough, gastrointestinal (GI) tract bleeding, frequent nausea and/or vomiting, persistent pain, iron-deficiency anemia, progressive unintentional weight loss, lymphadenopathy, epigastric mass, new-onset atypical symptoms at age 45 to 55 years (a lower age threshold may be appropriate, depending on local recommendations), and family history of either esophageal or gastric adeno-carcinoma. Answer choices B and D are incorrect, as these are typical GERD symptoms. Answer choice C is incorrect, as symptoms often worsen when lying flat and thus may result in nighttime awakening and the need to sleep with additional pillows to elevate the head of the bed or sleep in a recliner.[1]

3. **Correct answer: C**
   Rationale: Medications known to worsen GERD symptoms include calcium channel blockers, anticholinergic medications, and nonsteroidal anti-inflammatory drugs (NSAIDs). Other medications such as potassium supplements, tetracycline, and bisphosphonates may cause upper GI tract injury and exacerbate reflux-like symptoms or reflux-induced injury. Answer choices A and B have not been known to worsen GERD symptoms. Answer choice D is used to treat GERD symptoms.[1]

4. **Correct answer: D**
   Rationale: Answer choice A is incorrect. Tolerance will not be increased by eating foods that worsen heartburn. Trigger foods that worsen heartburn should be identified and avoided. Answer choice B is incorrect, as it is recommended to eat small meals throughout the day. Answer choice C is incorrect. It is advisable to avoid lying down for 2 hours after eating. This decreases the amount of stomach acid available for reflux.[1]

5. **Correct answer: A**
   Rationale: The patient has frequent symptoms more than 2 days a week thus it would be appropriate to try a 2-week trial of a PPI medication such as omeprazole. Answer choices B and C are incorrect, as the use of antacids and lifestyle changes would be insufficient for his symptoms based on severity and frequency. They will likely result in an impartial response but could be used in combination with other therapy, such as PPI. Answer choice D is incorrect, as the patient does not present with any alarm symptoms that would warrant a physician referral. Additionally, he tried Pepcid for his symptoms for nearly a week, but he has been taking them as needed for heartburn rather than schedule dosing 20 mg once or twice daily.[1]

6. **Correct answer: D**
   Rationale: After a 2-week trial of a PPI purchased over the counter, if symptoms return and may not be alleviated by lifestyle changes, you should refer the patient to the physician. Most patients will require a formal course of PPI therapy of adequate duration (usually 8 weeks) to assess the treatment response in GERD patients. Additionally, physicians want to ensure there is not an alternative diagnosis such as peptic ulcer disease, upper GI malignancy, functional dyspepsia, eosinophilic esophagitis, or cardiologic causes. Answer choice A is incorrect, as the patient has already completed a 2-week trial, and now they must be referred to a physician. Answer choice B is incorrect, as the patient stated the PPI helped reduce his symptoms but did not provide complete resolution and thus he will likely need a long-term PPI based on his symptom frequency and severity. Additionally, cimetidine is not the preferred

H2RA, as it has many drug interactions. Answer C is incorrect, as the use of antacids would be insufficient.[1,2]

7. **Correct answer: D**
   Rationale: When conducting a medication reconciliation for a patient, it is important to devise a best possible medication history (BPMH). This entails using multiple sources, including patient interview to assess what medications they are taking and how they are taking them, evaluation of the medication list in the EHR, contacting the patient's pharmacy(ies) where they fill their prescriptions to see what they are taking and how often they pick up their prescriptions, discharge medication list, and patient lists they may have. Often in the patient interview we gather meaningful information such as their adherence, and non-prescription medications they are taking. Once we get the BPMH, we can then perform a medication reconciliation to determine therapy recommendations for the patient.

8. **Correct answer: B**
   Rationale: Patients may not recall their medication history, and we must rely on other sources such as community pharmacy records, physician records, and patient or caregiver interviews. It is important to know what the patient has tried in the past, what worked, and what did not work when trying to devise a therapy plan for an acute problem. Answer choices A, C, and D are incorrect, as they are unlikely to result in accuracy of the medication record. Patients may try to guess what medications they were taking, but it is important for us to verify the information if possible through pharmacy or physician records.

9. **Correct answer: B**
   Rationale: PPI therapy is a risk factor for *C. difficile* infection in patients and should be used with caution in patients at risk. Answer choice A is incorrect, as short-term use of a PPI increases the risk for community-acquired pneumonia. This risk does not appear elevated in long-term use. Answer choice C is incorrect. GERD is a potential cofactor in patients with asthma, chronic cough, and laryngitis. PPI use does not increase risk of these conditions in patients with GERD. Answer choice D is incorrect. Long-term PPI use is permissible in patients with osteopenia and osteoporosis. In patients with osteoporosis and additional risk factors for hip fracture, we should caution long-term PPI use. Vitamin B_{12} deficiency and hypomagnesemia have also been associated with long-term PPI use.[2]

CASE 5

1. **Correct answer: E**
   Rationale: Identifying nonadherence and addressing barriers which contribute to poor compliance is important in optimizing medication therapy. If our patient has an educational deficit or a financial barrier that will prevent him from taking his prescribed medications correctly, our interventions will focus on addressing adherence and supporting our patient in resolving those financial barriers. Poor diet and lifestyle, including smoking, can also contribute to readmission and can be addressed when providing patient education. When reconciling medications, we should discontinue medications that can cause adverse effects for our patients, such as NSAIDs for patients with high blood pressure or cardiovascular events.

2. **Correct answer: A**
   Rationale: For this patient, cost is the major barrier. Our patient has Medicaid, states that he skips medication doses to prolong his refill and complains about lack of funds to pay for his medications. There are no apparent issues of forgetfulness or transportation issues, although these are important to address if they are a barrier to a patient. There is also no indication that the patient feels there is a lack of benefit. He skips doses due to cost.

3. **Correct answer: D**
   Rationale: How we address adherence issues will depend on the unique and individual needs of the patient. In this case, because cost is the primary issue, interventions should focus on identifying resources to support the patient in affording his medications. This may require collaboration with case management and social work. Interventions can include changing his medications to cheaper alternatives, ensuring his insurance covers prescribed medications, and identifying resources for supplemental funding. Although the other interventions are valuable, they will not address his adherence issue.

4. **Correct answer: D**
   Rationale: In patients with acute coronary syndrome treated with dual antiplatelet therapy after bare metal stent or drug-eluting stent implantation, P2Y12 inhibitor therapy (clopidogrel, prasugrel, or ticagrelor) should be given for at least 12 months along with aspirin 81 (75–100) mg daily. It is reasonable to use ticagrelor in preference to clopidogrel for P2Y12 treatment in patients with NSTE-ACS who undergo an early invasive or ischemia-guided strategy.[1,2]

5. **Correct answer: E**
   Rationale: Patients with an NSTEMI should be prescribed a beta blocker and an ACEi/ARB for mortality benefit. Nitroglycerin should be prescribed for symptomatic relief, with appropriate education provided. A high intensity statin should be prescribed for secondary prevention. Since cost is a major concern for our patient, we can support him in affording his medications, but it is important to also appropriately educate him on how these medications help him, why they are important, and why adherence is essential.[1,2]

6. **Correct answer: A**
   Rationale: The guidelines recommend risk reduction strategies for secondary prevention, which includes all eligible patients with NSTE-ACS should be referred to a comprehensive cardiovascular rehabilitation program either before hospital discharge or during the first outpatient

visit. The pneumococcal vaccine is only recommended for patients 65 years of age and older and in high-risk patients with cardiovascular disease. Although our patient was in pain upon admission, we do not need to refer him to a pain management specialist; however, we do need to ensure he understands he needs to stop taking Aleve, which is an NSAID for acute pain. The ACC/AHA guidelines state NSAIDs (except aspirin) should not be initiated and should be discontinued during hospitalization for NSTE-ACS because of the increased risk of major adverse cardiac events (MACE) associated with their use. Home healthcare can be a great intervention for patients to ensure they receive the care they need once returning home, but in this patient it is not necessary. The majority of this patient's barriers to care are cost related, adherence related, and a lower health literacy that leads to misunderstanding the importance of medications, how to take them, how they work, and what to expect.[1,2]

7. **Correct answer: A**
   Rationale: Early request for a prior authorization of ticagrelor for the patient would have given the physician time to fill out the necessary paperwork and allowed the insurance company time to process it. Comprehensive discharge planning and care coordination with case management and social work can help prevent issues like this by sending the prescription in advance of discharge and ensuring prior authorization is initiated while the patient is still in the hospital. This is an important intervention to reduce the risk of readmission if the patient is not adherent due to cost issues.

8. **Correct answer: A**
   Rationale: Early follow-up with patients after they return home from the hospital is a key clinical activity that can help identify patient risks that may lead to readmission. If the patient had been called 1 to 2 days after discharge, they would have recognized that DAPT after PCI with a DES is critical and the antiplatelet medication could be life sustaining. Options include changing the prescription to clopidogrel, which is not the preferred agent but would suffice and is relatively inexpensive. Other options include providing the patient with the manufacturer coupon card, initiation of prior authorization immediately upon receipt of the prescription, and helping the patient to explore patient assistance programs.

CASE 6

1. **Correct answer: C**
   Rationale: If the primary care provider realized that the patient struggled with the cost, he could have made appropriate adjustments in the medication to help reduce cost (e.g., combination therapy or utilizing a generic alternative). Although the patient did not have a home blood pressure monitor, a blood pressure monitor was readily available for use at his work. The only other home

medication that the physician may have not been aware of was the men's multivitamin. This medication does not impact the patient's blood pressure. This patient consumes well below the daily dietary recommendations for alcohol and caffeine (<2 alcoholic drinks per day for men; <400 mg of caffeine per day).

2. **Correct answer: C**
   Rationale: The Joint Commission promotes training, education, and coaching to reinforce successful hand-off techniques.[3] Information communicated to other healthcare providers should be standardized; customizing communication templates can lead to confusion and misunderstanding. In this case, if the hospital had communicated with the community pharmacy to obtain a medication list with refill history it would be apparent that the patient was not adherent to his medications. Adherence needs to be addressed prior to initiation of a new therapy or intensification of an existing therapy. Information should be relayed in a clear manner, so it may not be appropriate to use excessive abbreviations.

3. **Correct answer: D**
   Rationale: SBAR has been highly utilized by the healthcare system as a template to provide clear communication.[4] Clinical health status can be assessed through thorough review of subjective and objective information obtained from the patient chart and interview. There are several tools available to estimate the risk of medication non-adherence (Morisky Scale, Medication Adherence Questionnaire, etc.), but the SBAR tool is not one. The AHRQ Health Literacy Measurement Tools and The Health Literacy Tool Shed are both resources to help assess health literacy.

4. **Correct answer: A**
   Rationale: The statements in answer A are describing introductory information regarding the patient. B is a recommendation regarding the patient's antidepressant therapy. The statement in C is providing background information regarding this patient. D is an assessment of the patient's anxiety and depression.[4]

5. **Correct answer: A**
   Rationale: This patient has at least three risk factors for low health literacy (male, African American, and non-high school graduate).[9] The patient is overall confused regarding his medications and how they work. In addition, the patient admitted that he has difficulty paying for his medications. The patient did not mention any issues with transportation or side effects.

6. **Correct answer: B**
   Rationale: A summary section can be used to reword key points of the handout and increase comprehension. Illustrations should be simple line drawings so they can be more easily recognized. Nonessential details and colors can distract the viewer. Information should be provided at a 5th grade level. Size 12 font should be used to be sure the patient can read the content. Bolding and varying color

and size of font can be used to highlight important information; however, this should not be used excessively.[10]

7. **Correct answer: C**

   Rationale: The literature shows that providing written and verbal directions is more effective than providing verbal communication alone.[11] Not providing education to the patient can lead to more confusion and frustration. While it is important to send medications to the community pharmacy, it can lead to medication therapy problems if not sent with an updated medication list. In addition to written instructions, patients should be provided with simplified verbal instructions that break down complex ideas.[12]

8. **Correct answer: A**

   Rationale: The patient's discharge information including paperwork, labs, etc. should be shared with the patient's healthcare providers, including pharmacists. Medical insurance is primarily used in the physician's office and hospital to bill for medical claims. Knowledge of family history of hypertension would not impact care provided by the community pharmacist. In the community pharmacy prescription insurance is used to bill for medications, not medical insurance. The patient's medication list is protected health information that is not permitted to be shared with family members, friends, or other persons unless prior consent has been provided.

CASE 7

1. **Correct answer: D**

   Rationale: Multimodal pain management approach is considered ideal for patients post-TKA. Answer A is incorrect because upon transitioning home, the IV PCA pump needs to be converted to a PO option. Answer B is incorrect as nonsteroidal anti-inflammatory agents like celecoxib should be avoided in existing CKD. Answer C is incorrect as high potency opioids like PO oxycodone are not necessary for the treatment of moderate pain (4/10). Therefore, the most ideal choice for pain control is a moderate opioid analgesic like tramadol (answer D).

2. **Correct answer: C**

   Rationale: *The American College of Chest Physicians (ACCP) 2012 Antithrombotic Therapy and Prevention of Thrombosis*, 9th edition guidelines recommend the following for total hip or knee arthroplasty: low-molecular-weight heparin; fondaparinux; dabigatran, apixaban, or rivaroxaban; low-dose unfractionated heparin; adjusted-dose vitamin K antagonist; aspirin (all Grade 1B) for a minimum of 10 to 14 days.[8] While Direct Oral Anticoagulants (DOACs) like apixaban and dabigatran may be appropriate options for ease of administration, drug–drug interactions such as that with phenytoin will result in a reduced DOAC efficacy, making answers A and B incorrect.[9] Enoxaparin 100 mg SQ q12h is a treatment dose and not appropriate for prophylaxis, making answer D incorrect. Based on patient's renal function, the correct choice is enoxaparin 30 mg SQ q12h.[9]

3. **Correct answer: C**

   Rationale: According to the US Preventive Services Task Force guidelines, routine use of low-dose aspirin or alternative agents like clopidogrel for primary prevention is not clearly supported based on benefits versus risk comparison in patients above age 70; additionally, she has no clinical indication (e.g., stent placement) for clopidogrel use. This makes answers A and B incorrect.[10] Using aspirin along with VTE prophylaxis increases risk of bleeding and therefore its discontinuation (answer C) is the best choice. Increasing its dose to 325 mg only further increases risk of bleeding, making answer D incorrect.

4. **Correct answer: D**

   Rationale: This patient is Spanish-speaking and therefore language dissonance must be avoided in any transitions of care. The US Census Bureau reports that 85% of foreign-born US residents speak a language other than English at home and 28.9% of these self-identify that their English-speaking ability is not good or not at all.[11] Language-discordant care between patients and their providers increases the risk for a variety of poor outcomes such as poor management of diabetes, medication nonadherence, lack of health education, and dissatisfaction with care.[3–7] The omission of providing language-appropriate verbal and written education can marginalize patients, causing miscommunications and breakdowns in follow-up. Not understanding proper directions for her VTE prophylaxis may result in poor adherence, which can lead to increased risk for clotting or bleeding, making answer D correct. The patient's husband is driving her home and the patient has Medicaid these are not identified barriers to her transition home and therefore answers B and C are incorrect. Lastly, patients with chronic kidney disease are not considered high-risk beneficiaries for reducing readmission by the Center for Medicaid and Medicare, making answer A incorrect.

5. **Correct answer: C**

   Rationale: Teach-back is an evidence-based intervention that improves patient–provider communication, patient health outcomes, and patient safety.[12,13] Although active listening, nonverbal communication interpretation and motivational interviewing have their uses in effective patient counseling, they will not identify a language discordance if one exists; therefore, answers A, B, and D are incorrect. The teach-back method is used for many different conditions and diseases and has shown promise in helping patients and caregivers avoid medical mistakes and can help identify language barriers.[14,15] Teach-back serves to ensure that the healthcare provider explains information clearly, and is not considered a test or quiz. Asking the patient or caregiver to explain in their own words what they should do post-discharge is a way to check for understanding and if needed, reinforcement or perhaps an alternative strategy for communication. This makes answer C correct.

6. **Correct answer: C**
Rationale: Utilizing effective transitions of care intervention components, which includes providing language assistance, can reduce hospital readmission rates and yield high patient satisfaction.[15,16] Federal regulations require that language assistance services must be provided by any entity that receives federal financial assistance; they must be free of charge, be accurate and timely, and protect the privacy and independence of an individual with limited English proficiency. Covered entities must take reasonable steps to provide meaningful access to each individual with limited English proficiency.[17] This makes answer C correct. Services listed in answers A, B, and D are not mandated by regulatory agencies.

7. **Correct answer: A**
Rationale: According to the Nondiscrimination in Health Programs and Activities Rule by the US Health and Human Services Department published in 2016, a covered entity must offer a qualified interpreter to an individual with limited English proficiency to provide oral interpretation and a qualified translator when translating written content in paper or electronic form.[17] This written material should be translated using culturally appropriate translations per the CMS Toolkit Guidelines for Culturally Appropriate Translation.[18] Therefore, answer A is correct. According to the National Council on Interpreting in Health Care, a "qualified interpreter is an individual who has been assessed and demonstrated a high level of proficiency in at least two languages and has the appropriate training and experience to interpret with skills and accuracy…"[19] Therefore the use of a mobile application, family member, or other hospital employee would not meet the requirement for a qualified interpreter, rendering answers B, C, and D incorrect.

8. **Correct answer: A**
Rationale: The interpreter, serving as a conduit for conversation, should be seated next to or slightly behind the patient inconspicuously; this makes answer A correct. When using an interpreter, the healthcare provider should address the patient directly and should speak in first person, using "I" statements and avoid "tell him/her" or "he/she said" statements, rendering answers B and D incorrect. Simultaneous translation is not a common practice in medical interpreting. The provider should allow for sentence-by-sentence interpretations by speaking in short sentences or short thought groups and only asking one question at a time.[16] Therefore answer C is incorrect.

9. **Correct answer: B**
Rationale: The option which ensures the most timely administration involves contacting the patient's community pharmacy to ensure continuity of care, making answer B correct. Home delivery and mail order would not provide the dose for 8 pm that evening; therefore, answers A and C are incorrect. Holding discharge should only be considered in circumstances where there is no option for medication administration post-discharge, rendering answer D incorrect.

CASE 8

1. **Correct answer: B**
Rationale: Potential barriers to medication adherence can be categorized as patient related or treatment related. Patient-related barriers include lack of motivation, depression, denial, cognitive impairment, substance or alcohol abuse, cultural or alternate beliefs, and low healthcare literacy. Treatment-related barriers may include complex treatment regimens, actual or the concern for potential side effects, inconvenience, cost of medications, and time management.[2,3] The patient is on greater than five medications that are taken multiple times a day, thus answer B is most likely the barrier. Lack of motivation and low education level are patient-related and not treatment-related barriers (rules out answers C and D). Cost is less likely to be the treatment-related barrier as most of the medications in his list are generic and the patient has a prescription plan (rules out A).

2. **Correct answer: D**
Rationale: There is no one optimal way to measure a patient's adherence. It is important to use multiple methods to clarify the medications, as each method has its advantages and disadvantages. For example, it is important to call the pharmacy get a prescription record to assess if he has picked up his new medications and refilled his old medications. However, this can be inaccurate since the patient has been in and out of the hospital multiple times. Pill count is an objective and easily measurable but can be susceptible to error, especially if patients mix up their pills, throw them out, or are hospitalized. In addition, pill counting does not give you information about the timing of the pills consumed by the patient. A patient questionnaire is very simple and useful but is dependent on patient's recollection.

3. **Correct answer: D**
Rationale: It is important to develop trust with your patient. Patient's may not be honest about their lifestyle and habits because often times they don't want to disappoint their doctors. Thus, keeping this in mind, providers must try their best to phrase questions and approach interventions in a nonjudgmental manner. This can help facilitate a more open conversation between the doctor and the patient.[2] Asking questions that are blunt and without a lead-in statement can deter patients from being truthful (answer B).

4. **Correct answer: C**
Rationale: Wrong answers have either combination of age, race, sex, and socioeconomic status; they have not been consistently associated as major predictors for nonadherence so they should not be the sole basis for decisions when evaluating interventions to improve adherence.[2] Treatment of asymptomatic disease such as hypertension and diabetes, side effects of medications such as frequent urination and fatigue, lack of insight into illness due to inadequate patient education, and complex regimen with multiple pills that are to be taken multiple times a day are major predictors in AN for nonadherence.

5. **Correct answer: A**

   Rationale: One of the most effective ways to improve dosing schedules is by simplifying medication regimens from multiple times a day to once daily, as this has been correlated with increased adherence rates.[4] The patient is still hypertensive and not at goal, so increasing the blood pressure medication dose would be the most appropriate action. Since the patient forgets to take the second dose of lisinopril, it would be appropriate to simplify the dosing and change it from twice daily to once daily. Once-a-day dosing will help maximize adherence. Adding a clonidine patch is not the most appropriate action since the patient takes his medications at least once daily and there is room to increase his current blood pressure medications without the need to add another agent (answer B). It would not be beneficial to switch the patient from one antidiabetic agent to another since the A1C is at goal, and since AN forgets to take his medications twice daily, having a twice-a-day medication is not optimal (answer C). Discontinuing the aspirin is not appropriate since the patient had recent stents (answer D).

6. **Correct answer: D**

   Rationale: All the adherence aids above have been proven to be helpful. Medication reminders such as pill boxes, pill cards, compliance packaging, or technology integration can be employed based on patient preference. Pill cards are small pocket cards that contain name, dose, indication, and instructions for morning, afternoon, evening, and nightly doses. Technological methods include automatic text messages or smartphone free medication adherence applications.[5] Having an electronic application and a pill card will help him to remember his medications. Having a pill box will be convenient since he is always on the road (as long as he is keeping the medications in a cool, dry place).

7. **Correct answer: B**

   Rationale: Answer B is correct because when using teach-back, open-ended questions are the best questions because they facilitate a conversation. Answer A is incorrect because it has medical jargon using words such as "hypertensive urgency" which can confuse a patient. Answer C is incorrect because it is a yes/no kind of an question that doesn't help with teach-back. Finally, answer D is not correct because it may make the patient feel that provider is rushed/annoyed.

CASE 9

1. **Correct answer: A**

   Rationale: Answers B, C, and D are correct statements. However, it is a common misconception that clinicians manage the patient's chronic disease state (answer A). In fact, providers only manage the condition during brief follow-up appointments, and patients manage the condition at all other times.[1]

2. **Correct answer: D**

   Rationale: The correct answer is D, which is a widely accepted definition of "adherence."[2] Answer A refers to "persistence" and is not routinely utilized terminology. Answer B refers to "concordance," which is a clinically accepted medical term addressing the shared decision-making process. Answer C is incorrect because adherence indicates a patient is actively involved in their care. The term "compliance" is still commonly used, however, because this term is often inappropriately used interchangeably with "adherence." The term "compliance" has been considered politically incorrect by some because it may imply that the patient should "follow the provider's orders."[1]

3. **Correct answer: B**

   Rationale: JW is aware of why he is not taking his medications, so he is demonstrating intelligent nonadherence and B is correct. However, he is not obstinately avoiding his medication, therefore A is incorrect. The patient does not have a condition that causes him to forget his medications, therefore C is incorrect. There is no such thing as unintelligent nonadherence, hence D is incorrect.[1]

4. **Correct answer: B**

   Rationale: Common risk factors for nonadherence include dementia, depression, homelessness, substance abuse, complex treatment regimen, and cultural beliefs, among others (correct answer B). Job instability (answer D) is a potential risk factor; however, he has been employed as a truck driver for about 30 years. Living alone (answer C) and having a diagnosis of hyperlipidemia (answer A) are not specific risk factors for suboptimal medication adherence.[1]

5. **Correct answer: A**

   Rationale: Common behavioral interventions include developing a routine, simplifying the medication regimen, minimizing the cost, tailoring the regimen to individual needs, confirming appropriate administration technique, rewarding patient success, increasing the frequency of patient contact, using adherence aids, and enlisting the support of others. In this case, JW is not utilizing a device so administration technique (correct answer A) is not a factor that needs to be addressed. He may benefit from using adherence aids such as pill organizers (answer B), simplifying his regimen by changing bid medications to once daily (answer D), and enlisting the support of others such as his partner (answer E). Answer C is an appropriate intervention because it would be beneficial to find ways to increase the frequency of contact with the patient.[1]

6. **Correct answer: C**

   Rationale: JW's carvedilol adherence is decreased by the frequency of dosing; therefore C is correct. He understands his disease state and medications enough to know that it is his furosemide causing the issue, therefore A is incorrect. Answer B would be correct for the furosemide but would be incorrect for carvedilol.[1]

7. **Correct answer: D**

   Rationale: JW's clinical findings include bilateral crackles and LE edema, indicating nonadherence. Patient has potassium supplementation that will assist with keeping potassium within normal limits, so B is incorrect. Dry mouth and constipation may also occur; however, these would not interfere with JW's truck driving; therefore, A and C are incorrect.[1]

8. **Correct answer: B**
Rationale: The correct answer is B as JW has HFrEF and needs a beta-blocker indicated for this disease state. C is also wrong for this reason. Amlodipine at higher doses may make the swelling worse and does not have survival benefit in HFrEF. Patient is already taking an ace-inhibitor, and adding an ARB would increase the risk of kidney dysfunction, therefore A is incorrect.[1]

9. **Correct answer: B**
Rationale: The correct answer is a weekly pill box (answer B). JW does not like to use his cell phone, so A is incorrect. Likewise, a dose counter lid would be too much technology for this patient, making D incorrect. C is incorrect because JW is on the road frequently, so a bedside alarm clock will not be of use to him.[1]

CASE 10

1. **Correct answer: C**
Rationale: Technically, there is no indication for alendronate on this patient's profile. Because of her age and the fact that she is a woman, it is likely that she does have osteoporosis, but this should be documented in the chart. There is no drug–drug interaction between lisinopril and alendronate so option A is incorrect. There is no drug–drug interaction between ranitidine and pantoprazole so option B is incorrect. The patient is on multiple medications for GERD; therefore, option D is incorrect.

2. **Correct answer: C**
Rationale: It is assumed that FP is running out of medication early by taking it more often than prescribed, because every time she refills her prescription, it is too early. Although option A may be appropriate since the patient can pay out of pocket for the medication if it is not covered through insurance, the prescription should not be refilled if the patient is taking this medication incorrectly. Option B is incorrect because it states that FP is not taking her medication at all; however, according to the daughter, she is taking the medication. Option D is incorrect as there is no indication that she is taking additional doses of alendronate to help with her stomach issues.

3. **Correct answer: B**
Rationale: FP has full bottles of lisinopril in her cabinet, indicating that she is not taking the medication as prescribed. FP did not mention anything about cost or insurance issues related to lisinopril, so options A and D are incorrect. Option C does not make sense since her blood pressure was uncontrolled and taking too much of her antihypertensive would have the opposite effect.

4. **Correct answer: A**
Rationale: The patient was not adhering to her lisinopril prescription, likely leading to uncontrolled hypertension. The PCP did not realize that her uncontrolled BP was due to noncompliance so he added amlodipine. If the patient begins to take both lisinopril and amlodipine, this could significantly lower her blood pressure; therefore, option D is incorrect. Although lisinopril can cause hyperkalemia, taking both lisinopril and amlodipine does not put the patient at risk of hyperkalemia, so option B is incorrect. Neither lisinopril nor amlodipine can cause rebound HTN, so option C is incorrect.

5. **Correct answer: B**
Rationale: FP has not been taking lisinopril because of the cough; therefore, lisinopril should be discontinued. Additionally, FP has been taking amlodipine 5 mg daily and her blood pressure is close to the goal of <130/80 mmHg. We can wait to adjust her dose at her next visit if necessary. Option A is not correct as the patient's BP is elevated if she does not have hypertension. Although limiting sodium intake is recommended, it is not necessary to put the patient on a strict low sodium diet since the issue with her elevated BP is due to her not taking lisinopril; therefore, option C is not correct. Option D is not correct since we do not need to add a second antihypertensive medication right now. Even if we were to add another antihypertensive medication, other first-line therapies would be more appropriate than metoprolol such as HCTZ.

6. **Correct answer: C**
Rationale: Option A is not correct because motivational interviewing should be positive. It is important to encourage the patient to take their medications as prescribed. Additionally, you are not addressing the patient's concern. Option B is not correct because there are limited data to suggest herbal medication will help lower BP. We also do not know what interactions it has with KP's other medications. Lastly, we don't know if amlodipine is cheaper than herbal medicines, and if it is, we are still not addressing the patient's concern. Therefore, option D is not correct.

7. **Correct answer: A**
Rationale: We know that herbal products may interact with medications; therefore, option A is correct, and C is incorrect. Option B is not correct as herbal medicines may be inexpensive, making her more compliant. Option D is not correct, as we do not know if all herbal medicines are "bad." In addition, we should be constructive when talking to the patient.

CASE 11

1. **Correct answer: C**
Rationale:
Medication reconciliation: Prior to admission, PJ was taking lisinopril and was also prescribed insulin degludec and

insulin aspart. The patient has AKI, likely secondary to dehydration from having DKA. PJ's lisinopril should be held until her AKI resolves. While in the ICU, the patient's DKA should be managed with insulin per the hospital's DKA protocol, rather than resuming her home insulin regimen, which she was not taking, and probably the reason why she presented with DKA in the first place. Answer choices A and D are incorrect because they contain lisinopril.

Insulin management: PJ has moderate-severe DKA, as evidenced by her blood glucose greater than 250 mg/dL, bicarbonate less than 10 mg/dL, pH 7.15, anion gap is 28 mEq/L, and her dehydration and lethargy.[1-3] Either intravenous regular insulin or subcutaneous insulin aspart would be appropriate to manage PJ's DKA. Previous studies have shown that there is no significant difference in outcomes between intravenous regular insulin versus subcutaneous rapid-acting insulin when combined with aggressive fluid management for mild or moderate DKA.[1-4] Per the ADA 2021 guidelines, patients with uncomplicated DKA may be treated with subcutaneous insulin in the ED or step-down units.[3] When deciding the type of insulin to use, the hospital's DKA protocol, physician preference, nurse availability, cost, and other factors should be considered. The continuous infusion insulin should be continued until the patient's hyperglycemic crisis has resolved, as indicated by a blood glucose <200 mg/dL, plus at least two of the following: serum bicarbonate ≥15 mEq/L, venous pH >7.3, and a calculated anion gap ≤12 mEq/L (i.e., "anion gap closes").[1]

Fluid selection: In hyperglycemic patients, the extra glucose increases the osmolality of the extracellular fluid (ECF), causing water to move out of cells and into the ECF, thus diluting the serum sodium concentration and making it appear that the patient's sodium is lower than what it actually is. For every additional 100 mg/dL glucose above the normal glucose (100 mg/dL), the sodium concentration falls by about 1.6–2.4 mEq/L, and thus you should calculate a corrected serum sodium for patients in hyperglycemic crisis: corrected sodium = measured sodium + [0.016 (serum glucose 100)].[5,6] Using PJ's ICU admission labs, PJ's corrected sodium is 136–137 mEq/L, which is within the lower range of normal. Therefore 0.45% NaCl, rather than 0.9% NaCl, would be most appropriate to administer because 0.9% NaCl would put PJ more at risk for developing hypernatremia.[1,2] Answer choice A is incorrect. Dextrose 5% in water (D5W) should be started once a patient's blood glucose is less than 200–250 mg/dL to prevent the patient from becoming hypoglycemic while on insulin therapy to manage their DKA.

Potassium repletion: A patient with DKA may have an initial elevated serum potassium due to their acidemia, hypertonicity, and insulin deficiency.[1,2] With fluid and insulin administration, the patient's serum potassium will decrease. Proactive administration of 20–40 mEq of potassium chloride for every liter of IV fluids is recommended to maintain a serum potassium between 4–5 mEq/L to prevent hyperkalemia.[1-3]

Sodium bicarbonate: Sodium bicarbonate is generally not given and is not routinely recommended due to several studies showing no difference in time to discharge or resolution of acidosis.[4] However, if a patient's serum pH is less than 6.9, you can consider administering sodium bicarbonate 100 mEq in 400 mL sterile water plus potassium chloride 20 mEq at a rate of 200 mL/h for 2 hours or sodium bicarbonate 50 mEq in 500 mL of 0.45% NaCl until the venous pH is >7.0.[1,3] Sodium bicarbonate may also be indicated in patients with DKA who develop a non-anion gap hyperchloremic acidosis. Since PJ's pH is greater than 6.9 and she does not have a hyperchloremic acidosis, sodium bicarbonate is not indicated at this time. Answer choice A is incorrect.

Prophylaxis: PJ is at mild-moderate risk of developing a VTE, per her IMPROVE and Padua prediction scores of 0 and 4, respectively (3 points = immobile; 1 point = hormonal therapy).[7] Initially, while she is acutely ill and immobile in the ICU, it is reasonable to recommend pharmacologic prophylaxis per the 2012 CHEST Guidelines for Prevention of VTE in Nonsurgical Patients,[8] including, enoxaparin 40 mg subcutaneous daily (CrCl is ~50 mL/min) or unfractionated heparin subcutaneous every 8 to 12 hours. Answers A and B are incorrect because her renal clearance is ~50 mL/min; thus, no renal dose adjustment (enoxaparin 30 mg subcutaneous daily) is necessary at this time. At this time, PJ is not at high risk for developing a stress ulcer and likely does not need stress ulcer prophylaxis.[9]

2. **Correct answer: C**
   Rationale: Per the ADA 2021 guidelines, patients with type 1 diabetes mellitus usually require a weight-based insulin dose of 0.4–1 units/kg/day.[4] Of note, the ADA 2021 guidelines also reference the 2016 Diabetic Emergencies practice guidelines, which recommends 0.5–0.7 units/kg/day for DKA patients with newly diagnosed diabetes mellitus.[3]

   Lower threshold: 0.4 units (54.5 kg) = 21.8 units insulin total daily dose (TDD)

   Higher threshold: 1 unit (54.5 kg) = 54.5 units insulin TDD

   To calculate the basal and bolus total doses, divide the TDD in half:

   Lower threshold: 21.8 units / 2 = 10.9 units basal insulin and 10.9 units total bolus insulin

   Higher threshold: 54.5 units / 2 = 27.3 units basal insulin and 27.3 units total bolus insulin

   To calculate the mealtime bolus insulin, divide the total bolus insulin by 3 (for breakfast, lunch and dinner):

   Lower threshold: 10.9 units / 3 = 3.6 units bolus insulin with meals

   Higher threshold: 27.3 units / 3 = 9 units bolus insulin with meals

   Of the answer choices provided, answer C would be the most appropriate. Though the patient's home regimen (answer B) falls within an appropriate weight-based range, it is unlikely that the hospital has insulin degludec on formulary, so this answer is less feasible. Answer D is an appropriate basal-bolus regimen in general, but it is not appropriate for this patient since it is above the higher threshold. Answer A is not an appropriate basal-bolus regimen since the basal insulin dose (24 units) is twice that of the bolus total dose (12 units). The basal and bolus total doses should be about equal so that the patient gets 50% of their TDD as basal insulin and 50% of their TDD as bolus insulin.

3. **Correct answer: A**
   Rationale: Alternative to using weight-based dosing insulin, you can also use a patient's continuous insulin infusion rate to calculate the patient's total daily insulin requirement.[10] There are multiple ways to do this. One way is to first identify a 6-hour period of when PJ's glucose was well controlled while on the insulin drip and add the total insulin PJ needed for that 6-hour period and multiply by 4 hours to get the total daily dose (TDD) of insulin. You could also calculate the average insulin infusion rate for the last 12 hours and multiply that by 24 hours to get the TDD.[11] Once you have calculated the patient's TDD, you can convert 60% to 80% of the daily infusion dose into subcutaneous insulin.[4,10]

   - For example, from 0400 to 0900, 0300 to 0800, 0200 to 0700, 0100 to 0600: 14 units over 6 hours × 4 = 56 units TDD
   - Take 60%–80% of TDD: 56 units (0.8) = 33.6 to 44.8 units
   - Divide in half to calculate the total basal and total bolus doses: 33.6 to 44.8 units / 2 = 16.8 to 22.4 units (so 16.8–22.4 units basal total and 16.8–22.4 units bolus total)
   - Divide the total bolus insulin dose by 3 to calculate the mealtime bolus dose: 16.8 to 22.4 / 3 = 5.6 to 7.7 units with each meal

   Of the answer choices provided, answer A (24 units basal, 8 units bolus) is the closest to the calculated doses. Answer C does not take into consideration the 60% to 80% conversion factor and the higher dosing may put PJ more at risk for developing hypoglycemia. A high-intensity sliding scale insulin with meals may be appropriate but the doses of insulin glargine in answers B and D are not appropriate.

4. **Correct answer: C**
   Rationale: Per the 2021 ADA Diabetes Care in the Hospital guidelines, long-acting subcutaneous insulin should be overlapped with the continuous insulin infusion by 2 to 4 hours to prevent rebound hyperglycemia or recurrence of ketogenesis (i.e., "reopening the anion gap").[3,4,10,11] It is a common mistake to forget to overlap the insulin infusion with the long-acting subcutaneous insulin, but this is necessary because the half-life of intravenous insulin regular is significantly shorter (<10 minutes) than the delayed onset of long-acting subcutaneous insulin (~1–2 hours).[3,12,13]

5. **Correct answer: B**
   Rationale: In an outpatient setting, per the ADA guidelines, for nonpregnant adults the preprandial plasma glucose target is 80–130 mg/dL and the 1- to 2-hour postprandial glucose target is <180 mg/dL.[4,14] Upon discharge it is important for all patients with diabetes to have a good understanding of their glycemic targets for preprandial, as well as 2-hour postprandial blood glucose measurements. This will help achieve favorable results when it comes to lowering A1c values and to minimizing the risk of microvascular and macrovascular complications due to diabetes mellitus. Of note, glycemic goals are different based on different settings. Per the 2021 ADA Diabetes Care in the Hospital guidelines, insulin therapy should be given for a serum glucose ≥180 mg/dL, and a glucose target range of 140–180 mg/dL is appropriate for most critically ill and non-critically ill patients.[4,14,15] The AACE/ACE guidelines state that outpatient glucose targets for nonpregnant adults are <110 mg/dL for fasting plasma glucose and <140 mg/dL for 2-hour postprandial glucose, as in answer A.[16] Answer C is incorrect because it includes old ADA recommendations for a preprandial BG target of 70–130 mg/dL. Answers C and D are incorrect per the most current ADA guidelines.

6. **Correct answer: D**
   Rationale: Pneumococcal polysaccharide vaccine (PPSV23) is recommended for adults 19 years and older who have diabetes.[16,17] At different transitions of care, especially upon discharging patients from the hospital, it is important to provide education about the importance of receiving all the necessary immunizations. Individuals with diabetes are at a high risk for influenza infection and for developing serious influenza complications which can result in hospitalization and sometimes even death. Annual vaccination against influenza is recommended for all people 6 months of age and older, especially for those with diabetes.[16,17] Patients with diabetes are also at an increased risk for pneumococcal disease and associated complications. Pneumococcal conjugate vaccine (PCV13) is recommended for adults 19 years and older with an immunocompromising condition (not including diabetes), cerebrospinal fluid leak, or cochlear implant.[18] Thus, answer B is incorrect. In general, the shingles vaccines are approved and recommended for patients 50 years and older, but this is irrespective of whether they have diabetes, so answer C is incorrect.[18] It is also important to point out that patients ages 18 through 59 years with diabetes should be vaccinated for hepatitis B.[16,17] PJ has completed the hepatitis B series, but still needs the annual seasonal influenza vaccine and PPSV23.

7. **Correct answer: B**
   Rationale: When reconciling medications prior to hospital discharge, pharmacists should create the best possible medication list based on the patient's active problems, changes to health status, and treatment plan during the hospitalization, and relevant labs. Pharmacists should evaluate prior-to-admission medications, inpatient regimens, and discharge medication lists, as well as consider barriers to adherence, such as misconceptions about the medications, educational deficits and cost issues. The providers held the lisinopril on admission due to an increase in serum creatinine but since the patient's AKI has resolved and she was taking it for her microalbuminuria, it is appropriate to resume her lisinopril once she is transferred to the medicine floor and continued upon discharge. The patient

was not adherent to her prior-to-admission insulin regimen, so it would not be appropriate to resume. She had a cost issue with insulin degludec, and she was not taking the insulin lispro 5 units. It would be most appropriate to continue her inpatient regimen for management of her diabetes. The patient does not have an indication for a statin due to her age and lack of atherosclerotic cardiovascular disease. Per the ADA 2021 guidelines, statins for primary prevention are indicated for patients with diabetes between the ages of 40 to 75 years old but can be considered for 20 to 39 years old in patients who have additional atherosclerotic cardiovascular disease.[19] Lastly, she has no indication for pantoprazole. Acid suppression agents, such as proton pump inhibitors and histamine-2 receptor antagonists, started for stress ulcer prophylaxis in the ICU should be discontinued when transitioning to the medicine floor and not continued outpatient. If a patient has an acid suppressive agent with no clear indication, it should be discontinued.

8. **Correct answer: B**
   Rationale: A structured and clear plan tailored to each patient upon discharge is important in order to avoid readmission and to help ensure medication adherence. Per the ADA 2021 guidelines, an outpatient follow-up visit with the primary care provider, endocrinologist, or diabetes educator within 1 month of discharge is advised for all patients experiencing hyperglycemia in the hospital.[4,16,17] If glycemic medications are changed, which is the case for PJ, or glucose control is not optimal at discharge, an earlier appointment (in 1–2 weeks) is preferred.[4] PJ's AKI has resolved on discharge and although she has microalbuminuria, this can be managed by either her primary care physician or her endocrinologist for now. Thus, seeing the nephrologist is not needed at this time. This makes answers A and D incorrect. PJ should see her primary care provider, endocrinologist, and diabetes educator in 1 to 2 weeks, as her glycemic medications have changed in the hospital and her glucose control is not optimal.

9. **Correct answer: D**
   Rationale: Hypoglycemia management and hypoglycemia awareness counseling must be addressed upon discharge from the hospital in order to prevent future ED and hospital readmissions, especially given the fact that patients with type 1 diabetes mellitus are at an increased risk for hypoglycemia. PJ should be educated about signs and symptoms of low blood sugar, as well as management of low blood sugar with fast-acting carbohydrates at the hypoglycemia alert value of 70 mg/dL or less.[16,17] In order to prevent readmission to the hospital (i.e., recurrence of DKA), PJ should be counseled about the importance of adherence to her medications, especially insulin. This may need to involve a discussion about treatment goals and the risks associated with poorly controlled diabetes, including micro- and macrovascular complications.[16,17] For patients of childbearing age, special attention should be paid to the review of the medication list for potentially harmful medications such as angiotensin-converting enzyme inhibitors,

angiotensin receptor blockers, and statins.[20] As PJ is of childbearing age, she should be educated about lisinopril being a potentially harmful drug in pregnancy, regardless of whether she is on birth control.

CASE 12

1. **Correct answer: B**
   Rationale: Levothyroxine should be administered consistently in the morning on an empty stomach, at least 30 to 60 minutes before food and should not be administered within 4 hours of calcium- or iron-containing products (e.g., multivitamins). AP is taking atorvastatin as prescribed once daily (it can be taken at any time). AP is taking dulaglutide correctly once weekly (can be taken irrespective to meals or time of day).

2. **Correct answer: C**
   Rationale: Thyroid dysfunction, B_{12} deficiency, and chronic amiodarone use are associated with neuropathy and need to be ruled out before determining if a patient has neuropathy of diabetic origin. Conversely, vitamin K does not need to be evaluated, as imbalances are not necessarily shown to have correlation to neuropathy.[2]

3. **Correct answer: B**
   Rationale: CAN is associated with signs and symptoms of abnormal blood pressure control, resting tachycardia, and orthostatic hypotension. Answers A, C, and D (syncope, resting tachycardia, and orthostatic hypotension, respectively) fall within the criteria of CAN and are therefore incorrect. Answer B can be due to neuropathy but does not fall within the criteria of CAN specifically. Answer B, anhidrosis (abnormal sweating), is a sudomotor complication. Therefore, the correct answer is B.[1]

4. **Correct answer: D**
   Rationale: All of the counseling points listed are appropriate to mention for patients prescribed gabapentin. Gabapentin may cause drowsiness and dizziness and alter mood. Abruptly discontinuing gabapentin may also increase the likelihood of seizures—patients should be advised to contact their provider so that they can be monitored while they slowly taper down the medication if it needs to be discontinued.

5. **Correct answer: A**
   Rationale: Answer C, esophageal dysfunction, usually leads to pyrosis (heartburn) and dysphagia (difficulty swallowing). Answer D, CAN, can lead to symptoms such as resting tachycardia, abnormal blood pressure regulation, and orthostatic hypotension. Although metformin may cause GI symptoms, the patient has been diagnosed with diabetes for almost 20 years. As metformin is the first-line agent for management of diabetes, these GI symptoms would most likely have occurred after initiation. Therefore, answer B is incorrect. Gastroparesis is a

type of neuropathy in which there is inappropriate gastric emptying. Common symptoms include postprandial vomiting, bloating, and nausea. GLP-1 agonists, such as dulaglutide (started in AP 2 months ago), often cause gastrointestinal ADRs such as nausea and vomiting. Therefore, gastroparesis and dulaglutide may be the most reasonable causes of AP's GI symptoms.[1,2]

6. **Correct answer: C**
   Rationale: Answers A, B, and D are not indicated as first-line for diabetic neuropathy. A is not correct, as tapentadol has limited efficacy, potential for abuse, and risk for other serious ADRs. B is not correct as amitriptyline only shows limited efficacy and puts the patient at higher risk for anticholinergic side effects. D, venlafaxine, is not correct even though it has a similar mechanism of action as duloxetine, a first-line agent. Venlafaxine has shown to not be as efficacious as duloxetine for the mitigation of neuropathy. Pregabalin and duloxetine have high rates of success (30–50%) for treating neuropathy and are both FDA approved for this indication. Therefore, answer C is the best choice.[1,2]

7. **Correct answer: B**
   Rationale: Answer A is not correct as duloxetine, along with pregabalin, is FDA approved for diabetic peripheral neuropathy. Answer C is not correct as this is typically a side effect of tramadol, tapentadol, and other opioid derivatives. Answer D is incorrect as duloxetine is usually recommended for use only once daily. Common adverse effects of duloxetine are insomnia, anorexia, or sexual side effects; therefore, B is the best answer.

8. **Correct answer: C**
   Rationale: According to the ADA 2020 Standards for Care,[1] gabapentin may be considered a first-line agent for patients with difficult socioeconomic situations and has a similar efficacy profile to that of pregabalin. Answers A, B, and D may be cheaper alternatives but have limited efficacy and run the risk of serious ADRs (i.e., respiratory depression and anticholinergic effects). Therefore, C is the best choice.[1]

9. **Correct answer: C**
   Rationale: Answer A is incorrect, as adjusting insulin would not necessarily affect the neuropathy as the blood glucose is only slightly higher than goal. Answer B is also incorrect. Metformin may lead to B_{12} deficiency and may indirectly lead to neuropathy; however, the most recent B_{12} levels are within normal limits. Answer D is incorrect as metoprolol succinate is not an antihyperglycemic and will not affect peripheral neuropathy. AP may be experiencing nausea, vomiting, and bloating as a side effect of dulaglutide or due to gastroparesis, a type of neuropathy. Dulaglutide is not recommended in patients with gastroparesis, and the ADRs may be a barrier to adherence.

10. **Correct answer: D**
    Rationale: Dapagliflozin is known to reduce A1c by 0.5% to 1.0% and has positive cardiovascular data. This would be ideal for AP. Answer C, semaglutide is another type of GLP-1 agonist (like dulaglutide) and would not be recommended for AP due to his gastroparesis and recent nausea, vomiting, and bloating. Insulin aspart could be used but is not necessarily the best option as oral options have not been exhausted and it involves adding another injectable that could increase risk of hypoglycemia. Pioglitazone may be an effective option for lowering A1c but has been known to cause weight gain and is not optimal for the patient's cardiac history.

CASE 13

1. **Correct answer: B**
   Rationale: Acute kidney injury is an abrupt decrease in kidney function, regardless of the cause.[1] This function can be captured by the evaluation of serum creatinine (SCr) and/or urine output (UOP). Various definitions of AKI have been developed, but there is a need for a unified definition to support clinical practice, research, and public health efforts. According to the KDIGO Clinical Practice Guidelines of Acute Kidney Injury, AKI is defined as:
   - An increase in SCr by ≥ 0.3 mg/dL within 48 hours; or
   - An increase in SCr to ≥ 1.5 times baseline which is known or presumed to have occurred within the prior 7 days; or
   - A urine volume <0.5 mL/kg/hr for 6 hours.

   AKI can be further staged based on severity using UOP and SCr. However, it must be remembered that both UOP and SCr are only surrogate markers of glomerular filtration rate (GFR). Staging is helpful in assessing the risk of short- and long-term complications and the need for renal replacement therapies.

2. **Correct answer: B**
   Rationale: While the kidney is a resilient organ, the risk of AKI is increased by i) factors that increase the susceptibility for developing AKI, and/or ii) exposure to factors that cause AKI.[1] It is the interplay between susceptibilities and exposures that determines the development of AKI. Susceptibility factors vary among patients and may be modifiable. KJ's susceptibility factors include dehydration/volume depletion, advanced age, female gender, African American ethnicity, CKD, and diabetes. While all these factors may have contributed, dehydration represents a change from baseline, is acute, and should be corrected.

3. **Correct answer: B**
   Rationale: Based on the assessment of a patient's susceptibility factors, exposures can be evaluated for their risk versus benefit.[1] Metformin, which is contraindicated in certain levels of reduced renal function, is not nephrotoxic on its own. For KJ, the exposure to an angiotensin converting enzyme (ACE) inhibitor (i.e., lisinopril), a

nonsteroidal anti-inflammatory drug (NSAID) (i.e., ibuprofen), and a diuretic (i.e., hydrochlorothiazide), in addition to her numerous susceptibility factors poses a significant risk for developing AKI.[2] While these agents are commonly prescribed together, they are potentially nephrotoxic as monotherapy and may have deleterious effects when combined.

4. **Correct answer: A**
   Rationale: It is important to understand the cause of AKI to provide targeted interventions, if available, and appropriate general supportive care. Prerenal AKI is the most common form of AKI.[2] This is caused by an alternation in renal hemodynamics that leads to reduced glomerular filtration pressure, reduced renal blood flow, or both. This results in a decline in GFR.

   Maintenance of renal hemodynamics requires an intricate system of autoregulation of blood flow, intraglomerular capillary hydrostatic pressure, GFR, and UOP.[2] Under normal conditions, autoregulation readily maintains renal blood flow and pressure. Simplistically, this system of autoregulation includes prostaglandin (PGE)-mediated afferent arteriole vasodilation and angiotensin II (ATII)-mediated afferent and efferent arteriole vasoconstriction to increase and maintain intraglomerular pressure and perfusion. In times of reduced renal blood flow and pressure, these neurohormonal mechanisms help sustain appropriate renal hemodynamics and prevent resultant damage to the renal tissues. However, if prerenal AKI is prolonged, damage may ensue.

   NSAIDs decrease cyclooxygenase mediated synthesis of vasodilatory prostaglandins (prostacyclin and prostaglandin E_2) which act on the afferent arteriole.[2] Similarly, ACE inhibitors reduce the synthesis and activity of ATII, resulting in dilation of the efferent arteriole. Both NSAID-induced afferent arteriole vasoconstriction or ACE inhibitor–induced efferent arteriole vasodilation can lead to reduced hydrostatic pressures, renal ischemia, loss of GFR, and AKI. However, when these two agents are combined, there is an even greater risk.

   Diuretics, often used to maintain volume status and blood pressure, can lead to hypotension and volume depletion.[2] These are susceptibilities for the development of AKI on their own. The body's natural compensatory mechanism to hypotension or hypovolemia, is activation of the renin-angiotensin-aldosterone system (RAAS). When diuretics are given in combination with an ACE inhibitor, these compensatory mechanisms are blunted or insufficient.

   While prolonged prerenal disease could progress to intrinsic disease, information obtained on the urinalysis would be markedly different, indicating renal tissue damage. Therefore, option B is incorrect. Acute tubular necrosis is a form of intrinsic renal injury; therefore, option C is incorrect. Option D is incorrect as obstructive disease is typically due to an obstruction of urine flow downstream from the kidney, and is resultant from an obvious cause.

5. **Correct answer: C**
   Rationale: KJ's estimated creatinine clearance (CrCl) is 23 mL/min (using the Cockcroft-Gault equation). KJ's current eGFR is 21 mL/min/1.73 m² using the CKD-EPI equation.[3] Metformin use is contraindicated in patients with eGFR less than 30 mL/min/1.73 m², so it should be discontinued at this time. Restarting metformin for outpatient use can be considered once the eGFR is 30 to 45 mL/min/1.73 m² (at 50% reduced dose) or above 45 mL/min/1.73 m² (full dose). Answer A is incorrect because glyburide is not recommended for use in patients with CKD or in older adults due to its prolonged half-life in renal impairment that may lead to hypoglycemia.[4,5] Answer B is incorrect because the use of antithrombotic doses of aspirin (75–162 mg/day) are recommended for cardiovascular risk reduction in patients with diabetes and CKD or dialysis patients.[6] Low-dose aspirin does not require dose reduction or discontinuation for KJ's CrCl.[3] Answer D is incorrect because changing metoprolol succinate to metoprolol tartrate would increase the frequency of administration from once to twice daily and potentially decrease medication adherence. Metoprolol (succinate or tartrate) does not require dose adjustment for renal insufficiency.[3]

6. **Correct answer: C**
   Rationale: Patients admitted to the hospital who take oral antidiabetic medications as outpatients should have oral medications discontinued with a transition to insulin therapy while hospitalized.[7] The preferred insulin regimens are basal insulin monotherapy or basal insulin plus bolus insulin (if eating) prior to meals. Answer A is incorrect because insulin is the preferred management strategy. Also, sulfonylureas are associated with hypoglycemia, especially in patients who are not eating. Answer B is incorrect because the sulfonylurea should be discontinued while KJ is hospitalized and because sliding scale insulin is strongly discouraged in clinical practice guidelines.[7] Answer D is incorrect because SGLT2 inhibitors are not recommended for routine inpatient use. Also, SGLT2 inhibitors are not recommended in patients with eGFR less than 30 mL/min/1.73 m².[3]

7. **Correct answer: D**
   Rationale: Although KJ was hypotensive upon hospital admission, her blood pressure was at goal (<130/80 mmHg) on home medications prior to admission.[6,8] KJ's blood pressure is not currently at goal, likely due to modifications in her home antihypertensive regimen during hospitalization. Now that KJ's SCr is back to baseline, restarting her home lisinopril/HCTZ regimen is the most appropriate first step to getting her blood pressure back to goal. According to clinical practice guidelines, thiazide diuretics and ACE inhibitors are first-line agents for hypertension treatment and are appropriate for patients with diabetes and CKD without albuminuria.[8] In patients with diabetes and CKD who have albuminuria, an ACE inhibitor is recommended first-line for hypertension treatment.[8] Restarting KJ's metoprolol succinate should

also be considered, as this was part of the home antihypertensive regimen that resulted in her blood pressure being at goal. Answers A and B are incorrect as KJ's A1c is above goal, so a decrease in medication dose is inappropriate. KJ's blood glucose of 90 mg/dL on admission was likely due to her recent decreased oral intake. However, she is now hyperglycemic and her A1c of 10% reflects uncontrolled blood glucose over the past 3 months.[9] Clinical practice guidelines recommend an A1c goal of <7% in most non-pregnant adults; however, a less stringent A1c goal (e.g., <7.5% or <8.0–8.5%) is recommended in older adults with certain comorbidities. Answer C is incorrect because the recommended dose of aspirin for cardiovascular disease risk management in patients with CKD and diabetes is 75 to 162 mg/day.[6] Answer E is incorrect because naproxen is a nonselective NSAID, like ibuprofen, that carries the same risk of AKI.[10]

8. **Correct answer: A**
   Rationale: Mild pain should be treated with non-opioid analgesics.[11] Acetaminophen is the non-opioid analgesic of choice in patients with CKD.[11] Because of NSAID effects on the kidney in general as well as KJ's recent experience with NSAID use contributing to AKI, this class of drugs should be avoided. Answer B is incorrect because systemic absorption and AKI have been reported with topical NSAIDs, such as diclofenac, making this a less desirable choice. Answer C is incorrect because COX-2 selective NSAIDs adversely affect renal function like nonselective NSAIDs.[10] Answer D is incorrect because non-opioid analgesics should be used to treat mild pain (pain scale 1–3). Opioids can be considered for treatment of moderate (pain scale 4–6) or severe (pain scale 7–10) pain.[11]

9. **Correct answer: B**
   Rationale: UOP and SCr are both used to evaluate acute changes in GFR; however, each has important considerations surrounding its use. Increases or decreases in SCr lag changes in GFR by 1 to 2 days.[1,12] This may significantly delay the diagnosis of AKI, impede appropriate dose adjustments of medications as AKI is progressing or resolving, and adversely affect patient outcomes. However, due to the ease of obtaining an SCr, trends in this laboratory value can be helpful in assessing resolution of AKI in the outpatient setting. Theoretically, changes in UOP can be observed immediately, are more reflective of GFR, and will capture more cases of AKI. However, obtaining a measure of UOP in the outpatient setting is impractical, making answer A incorrect.

   It is important to have an estimate of a patient's baseline renal function in the form of an eGFR or an estimated CrCl to allow for monitoring trends, progression in chronic disease, and appropriate dosing of medications.[12] However, estimation of GFR or CrCl have several considerations. First, patients with unstable kidney function present a unique situation because SCr concentration values are changing, and steady state cannot be assumed. Both methods assume steady-state concentrations of SCr; therefore, their utility in evaluating patients with AKI is limited. These equations typically overestimate GFR when AKI is worsening and underestimate it when the AKI is resolving. Second, equations such as the MDRD and Cockcroft-Gault were developed for the purpose of identifying and stratifying CKD based on large multicenter epidemiologic studies and individualizing medication dosage regimens in patients with acute and chronic kidney disease, respectively. Extrapolation of their use in the setting of AKI requires additional research, making options C and D incorrect.

10. **Correct answer: D**
    Rationale: Studies (mostly observational) have linked PPIs to several adverse effects, such as *C. difficile* infection, fractures and bone loss, kidney injury, and nutritional deficiencies.[13,14] These adverse effects are of particular concern in older adults. Answer A is incorrect because KJ does not report GERD symptom on her current famotidine therapy. If she did have persistent symptoms despite adequate H2RA treatment, this would support the change to a PPI. Answer B is incorrect because PPIs are more potent inhibitors of gastric acid secretion than H2RAs. Answer C is incorrect because PPIs, not H2RAs, have been associated with fractures and bone loss.[15]

CASE 14

1. **Correct answer: D**
   Rationale: The three laboratory tests listed above are cardiac biomarkers, and elevations in these are used by clinicians to help diagnose acute coronary syndrome (ACS). Creatinine kinase (CK) is an enzyme released by nonspecific muscle cell necrosis or death. CK is first detectable about 4 to 6 hours after insult and remains detectable for about 2 to 3 days. CK-MB is a component of CK and is more specific to cardiomyocytes. When cardiomyocyte necrosis occurs, CK-MB is detectable in about 3 to 4 hours and remains elevated for about 1 to 2 days. Troponin is a protein found in heart (and skeletal) muscle. Troponin I and T are cardiospecific, and elevated levels indicate cardiomyocyte necrosis. Troponins become detectable about 3 to 4 hours after insult and can remain elevated for up to 14 days. Other laboratory tests that may be useful in diagnosis of ACS are myoglobin, BNP, NT-proBNP, alk phos, AST, and LDH.

2. **Correct answer: C**
   Rationale: The patient presented with chest discomfort at rest and has several coronary artery disease (CAD) risk factors: age, sex, HTN, dyslipidemia, DM, overweight, sedentary job, family history. His atherosclerotic cardiovascular disease (ASCVD) risk score prior to the event was 34.3%. This indicates high risk. His EKG revealed t-wave inversions indicating myocardial ischemia, and his biomarkers

are positive for myocyte necrosis (CK, CK-MB, and cTnT are all elevated). In combination, this points to NSTEMI. If his EKG had revealed ST-segment elevations, this would have indicated STEMI. If his biomarkers were negative, his likely diagnosis would have been unstable angina.

3. **Correct answer: B**
Rationale: Unless contraindicated (e.g., allergy), all patients with suspected ACS should be given an aspirin loading dose of 162 to 325 mg PO (chewed) as early as possible.[1] Prior to catheterization, patients should also be loaded with clopidogrel 300 to 600 mg, prasugrel 60 mg, or ticagrelor 180 mg.[1] The patient should then continue on ASA 81to 325 mg PO daily for life and a dual antiplatelet maintenance regimen (ASA + additional antiplatelet agent) for at least 12 months.[1] ASA doses greater than 162 mg offer no additional protection and increase risk of bleeding.[1] The additional antiplatelet agent could be clopidogrel 75 mg PO daily, prasugrel 10 mg PO daily, or ticagrelor 90 mg PO bid.[1] The 2014 guidelines note that it is reasonable to prefer ticagrelor or prasugrel over clopidogrel in patients who undergo invasive strategies (e.g., catheterization and stenting).[1] There are a few caveats to these regimens. If ticagrelor is chosen, the dose of daily ASA should not exceed 100 mg daily as higher doses can render the ticagrelor ineffective. Prasugrel should be avoided if the patient has a history of stroke, age $\geq$75 years, or a body weight of <60 kg.

4. **Correct answer: A**
Rationale: Beta-blocker use is part of the Centers for Medicare and Medicaid (CMS)/Joint Commission Acute Myocardial Infarction Core Measure Set. These measures must be documented in the patient medical record and are subject to audit by CMS and the Joint Commission. Beta-blockers decrease HR and contractility thereby decrease cardiac oxygen demand. Patients presenting with NSTEMI should be started on a beta-blocker within 24 hours of admission as this drug class has been shown to prevent fatal arrythmias triggered by ischemia.[1] It is preferred to start with a short acting agent dosed frequently in the acute setting. Once the patient is stable, transition to a long-acting agent is appropriate. PO beta-blockers are generally preferred to IV.[1] IV beta-blockers increase the risk of shock in patients with risk factors (age >70 years, HR >110 bpm, systolic BP <120 mmHg, and late presentation).[1] Beta-blockers should not be started in patients that present with concurrent HF (e.g., LEE, pulmonary edema, low EF, etc.).[1] Having DM is not a contraindication for beta-blocker use. It may decrease the patient's ability to sense hypoglycemia, and the patient should be educated about this possible effect and how to mitigate it.

5. **Correct answer: A**
Rationale: The patient now has documented clinical ASCVD; this necessitates high intensity statin therapy (>50% reduction in LDL-C) and trying to attain a goal LDL-C of <70 mg/dL.[2] There is no known benefit to adding ezetimibe at this time. He should be maxed on statin before adding another agent. He does have a slightly elevated AST, but this is likely due to the NSTEMI. AST is non-specific and can be elevated in ACS events. The ALT is WNL. This is not of concern in this situation. Elevations in liver enzymes of >3 × ULN do warrant concern, and if the patient is on a statin, it should be stopped.

6. **Correct answer: C**
Rationale: NSAIDs are contraindicated in post-ACS patients as these can render ASA not effective due to reversible platelet inhibition.[1] NSAIDs can also increase BP and fluid retention and are associated with an increased risk of CV events.[1] Option A is incorrect as NSAIDs are the mainstay therapy for OA, not APAP.[3] As for option B, although there is an interaction between NSAIDs and ticagrelor (increased risk of bleeding), concomitant use of the two classes of medications are not contraindicated. It should be used with caution and patients should be monitored for signs/symptoms of bleeding.

7. **Correct answer: A**
Rationale: Glucosamine and turmeric can increase the risk of bleeding so it should be avoided since KT is on aspirin and ticagrelor (and an SSRI). Thus, all the other options are incorrect. Additionally, according to the ACR/AF guideline, glucosamine is strongly recommended against in patients with knee OA as there is a lack of evidence to support use of glucosamine in patients with OA.[3]

8. **Correct answer: B**
Rationale: SSRIs have antiplatelet properties so sertraline may enhance the antiplatelet effect when taken concomitantly with an antiplatelet agent. Change in medication is not warranted; however, signs and symptoms of bleeding should be monitored. Option A is incorrect because SSRIs do not decrease the levels of ticagrelor. Option C is incorrect because ticagrelor does not decrease the effectiveness of SSRIs. Option D is incorrect because ticagrelor does not inhibit the metabolism of sertraline.

9. **Correct answer: C**
Rationale: ACE inhibitors reduce mortality in patients with recent MI and should be continued indefinitely in all patients with hypertension and/or diabetes mellitus.[1] As such, options A, B, and D are not correct. KT does not have a strong indication to continue HCTZ so it may be discontinued as long as the BP is adequately controlled with other antihypertensive medications. Lisinopril and HCTZ comes as a combination product so this would be another option to simplify the patient's antihypertensive medications.

CASE 15

1. **Correct answer: C**
Rationale: As patients with T2DM are often converted to insulin therapy upon hospital admission, it is important

to evaluate the safety, efficacy, and feasibility of their home antihyperglycemic regimens when preparing for discharge. In 2008, the United States Food and Drug Association (US FDA) began requiring that pharmaceutical companies demonstrate that antihyperglycemic agents used in the treatment of T2DM do not result in increased cardiovascular (CV) risk in what were dubbed CV Risk Outcomes Trials (CVOTs).[1] This call for action was spurred by events exhibited with use of rosiglitazone. Thiazolidinediones, such as rosiglitazone and pioglitazone, can exacerbate heart failure (HF) due to their potential to increase fluid retention. This side effect results from their ability to cause peripheral vasodilation as well as reduction of sodium and water excretion secondary to insulin sensitization at the renal level. Thiazolidinediones are contraindicated in persons with New York Heart Association (NYHA) Class III–IV HF and should be used with caution in persons with Class I–II HF.[2,3] It will be important to relay the importance of why this medication has been discontinued to AK, as well as communicate this change to his outpatient provider managing his T2DM.

Dapagliflozin is a sodium-glucose transporter-2 inhibitor (SGLT2i) that demonstrated no increased risk of major adverse CV event (MACE) outcomes compared to placebo in the DECLARE-TIMI 58 trial. However, it did demonstrate reduced potential for HF exacerbations and CV death compared to placebo in those without T2DM with NYHA Class II–IV HFrEF on guideline-directed medical therapy (GDMT), per results of the DAPA-HF trial.[3] Provided AK's renal function remains stable and he is not volume depleted, restarting dapagliflozin at discharge would be beneficial for both glycemic control and HFrEF once he is appropriately titrated to GDMT.

The biguanide, metformin, is unlikely to exacerbate AK's HF, and poses no additional CV risk. Rare cases of lactic acidosis have been reported in persons utilizing metformin suffering from tissue hypoperfusion states, such as acute decompensated HF. However, restrictions for use of metformin in patients with HF were redacted by the US FDA in 2006 due to evidence that its use in HF resulted in better therapeutic outcomes compared to patients on alternative regimens.[3] Provided the patient's HF and renal function remain stable, metformin may be safely restarted in the outpatient setting.

Semaglutide is a glucagon-like-peptide-1 agonist (GLP1a) that has demonstrated utility in improving glycemic control as well as reducing CV risk in persons with preexisting CV disease, per the results of PIONEER-6.[3] Given the patient's history of CAD, previous MI, and HF, continuation of semaglutide at discharge would be beneficial and would not increase his risk of HF exacerbation. The patient's dose of semaglutide could potentially be titrated further in the outpatient setting if he experiences glycemic dysregulation upon discontinuation of rosiglitazone.

2. **Correct answer: D**
Rationale: Bisoprolol is one of the three beta-blockers that has demonstrated efficacy in reducing morbidity and mortality in patients with HFrEF (Table 15-1). Bisoprolol, carvedilol, and metoprolol succinate should be preferentially prescribed in patients with HFrEF, and if patients are maintained on alternate beta-blockers, they should be switched to one of these three agents. The dose recommended for bisoprolol in this is approximately equivalent to the dose of propranolol that the patient was taking prior to admission. Starting bisoprolol at an equivalent dose to his propranolol will prevent regression in titrating to target doses known to demonstrate benefit based on the results of the CIBIS II trial.[4,5] As his propranolol is being switched to an alternate beta-blocker, it will be essential to relay this to AK, as well as his outpatient providers, to prevent possible duplication of therapy if his propranolol his restarted or is re-prescribed, in conjunction with his new bisoprolol.

Use of metoprolol tartrate is not recommended for patients with HF due to the lack of compelling evidence for its use. If use of metoprolol is desired based on cost, formulary, or patient preferences, metoprolol succinate would be preferred based on data demonstrating benefit in reducing morbidity and mortality at target doses in those with HFrEF based on the results of the MERIT-HF study.[4,5]

Carvedilol is an evidence-based beta-blocker that has demonstrated benefit in reducing morbidity and mortality at target doses in those with HFrEF based on the results of the COMET trial. However, the dose recommended above should only be considered in patients >85 kg who have previously tolerated standard target doses of carvedilol at 25 mg bid, which eliminates it as an option. Pharmacists should not only assess the appropriateness of a particular agent when a patient is moving from one level of care to another, but also if dosing is both safe and effective.[4,5]

Propranolol is not one of the three beta-blockers that has demonstrated evidence in reducing morbidity and mortality in HF, so continuing this agent upon discharge is not appropriate.[4,5]

3. **Correct answer: C**
Rationale: Patients should be instructed to monitor their weight on a daily basis as an indicator of fluid loss or retention. Patients should be advised that if they gain >2 to 3 pounds in 1 day or >5 pounds in 1 week that they should contact their healthcare provider or follow a medication action plan for further direction. In conjunction with this, it is essential to provide education on the role of diuretics in the symptomatic management of HF.[4,5]

Sodium restriction is recommended for all HF patients, but the amount that can be ingested per day differs depending on the degree of disease severity. In patients with American Heart Association (AHA) Stage A/B HF, sodium should be restricted to <1.5 g daily. In patients with AHA Stage C/D HF, sodium should be restricted to <3 g daily.

TABLE 15-1. Evidence-Based Beta-Blockers[4,5]

Medication	Initial Dose	Target Dose
Bisoprolol	1.25 mg daily	10 mg daily
Carvedilol	3.125 mg bid	25 mg bid*
Metoprolol succinate	12.5–25 mg daily	200 mg daily

*Doses of carvedilol 50 mg bid can be trialed in those >85 kg tolerating carvedilol 25 mg bid.

Data suggest that in patients with excessive sodium intake, defined as ≥3.8 g per day, the risk of acute HF exacerbation increases, making answer A incorrect.[4–6]

Current guidelines recommend restricting fluid intake to 1.5 to 2 L per day in patients with AHA Stage D HF, particularly if comorbid hyponatremia is present, as this has been shown to reduce the risk of hospitalization due to acute HF exacerbation. The parameters to restrict fluid intake to <0.5 L per day has not been shown to improve outcomes and can potentially lead to dehydration with use of diuretic agents, making answer B incorrect.[4,5,7]

Answer D is incorrect, as routine exercise has been shown to not only increase quality of life in HF patients but reduce subsequent hospitalizations. Current guidelines recommend exercise training in all patients with HF following testing to determine suitability of activities and ensure complicating comorbid conditions are not present.[4,5,8]

4. **Correct answer: B**
   Rationale: Table 15-2 lists the intensities of various statin regimens.

   AK is currently managed with a moderate-intensity statin dose. All patients with a history of clinical atherosclerotic CV disease (ASCVD) should be managed with a high-intensity statin to appropriately reduce CV risk, provided they are able to tolerate such doses and have an adequate life expectancy to receive benefits of use. Providers should target a reduction in low-density lipoprotein cholesterol (LDL-C) of >50% or, in very high-risk patients like AK, reducing LDL-C to a goal of <70 mg/dL. Table 15-3 illustrates very-high-risk characteristics that can increase the likelihood of recurrent CV events, justifying intensification of LDL-C reduction goals.[9]

   Answer A is incorrect, as he is currently receiving a moderate-intensity statin dose, as noted in Table 15-2. While this dose will still impart pleiotropic benefits known to statins, such as atherosclerotic plaque stabilization, reduced endothelial dysfunction, and inhibition of inflammatory responses, it is unlikely to provide the LDL-C reduction desired to reduce CV risk. This choice could be considered if AK had a life expectancy of <3 to 5 years or if he had previously been intolerant of high intensity statin regimens, but his medical history gives no indicator of those factors.[9]

TABLE 15-2. Statin Intensities[9]

High-Intensity Statin (expected LDL-C reduction >50%)	Moderate-Intensity Statin (expected LDL-C reduction 30%–50%)	Low-Intensity Statin (expected LDL-C reduction <30%)
Atorvastatin 40–80 mg	Atorvastatin 10–20 mg	Simvastatin 10 mg
Rosuvastatin 20–40 mg	Rosuvastatin 5–10 mg	Pravastatin 10 mg
	Simvastatin 20–40 mg	Lovastatin 20 mg
	Pravastatin 40–80 mg	Fluvastatin 20–40 mg
	Lovastatin 40 mg	Pitavastatin 1 mg
	Fluvastatin XL 80 mg	
	Fluvastatin 40 mg bid	
	Pitavastatin 2–4 mg	

LDL-C, low density lipoprotein cholesterol

TABLE 15-3. Very-High-Risk Characteristics for Future ASCVD Events[9]

Major ASCVD events
ACS with past 12 months
History of MI
History of ischemic stroke
Symptomatic peripheral arterial disease (claudication with ABI <0.85, revascularization, amputation)
Age ≥ 65 years
Heterozygous familial hypercholesterolemia
History of prior CABG or PCI interventions outside of ACS
Diabetes mellitus
Hypertension
CKD (eGFR 15–59 mL/min/1.73 m²)
Current smoker
LDL-C ≥100 mg/dL despite maximally tolerated statin therapy + ezetimibe
History of HF

ASCVD, atherosclerotic cardiovascular disease; ACS, acute coronary syndrome; MI, myocardial infarction; ABI, ankle brachial index; CABG, coronary artery bypass graft; PCI, percutaneous coronary intervention; CKD, chronic kidney disease; eGFR, estimated glomerular filtration rate; LDL-C, low density lipoprotein cholesterol; HF, heart failure

Answer C is incorrect, as ezetimibe should not be considered as an additive therapy until AK is optimized on a high-intensity statin dose, or unless AK is unable to achieve an LDL <70 mg/dL with a maximally tolerated statin dose if he experiences side effects with high-intensity therapy. The same holds true for answer D. It should also be noted that trials studying the proprotein convertase subtilisin/kexin type 9 inhibitors (PCSK9i), alirocumab and evolocumab, excluded persons with NYHA class III–IV HF from enrollment, so the benefit of their use in these populations is questionable.[9]

5. **Correct answer: C**
Rationale: Loop diuretics such as furosemide inhibit sodium-potassium-chloride cotransporters in the ascending loop of Henle, resulting in increased excretion of these specific ions. Because of this mechanism, loop diuretics are often referred to as "potassium wasting" diuretics. Serum potassium should be monitored with the use of loop diuretics, though in some cases their potassium wasting effects may be counterbalanced by medications affecting the renin-angiotensin-aldosterone system (RAAS) commonly used in HF. In situations where this is not the case, potassium supplementation can be used to replete and/or maintain potassium levels. Serum potassium should be reassessed at his outpatient follow-up appointment to ensure levels are appropriate. AK should also be educated on the reason why he has been prescribed potassium supplementation and which medications he is taking that could possibly affect his serum potassium levels.[5,6]

Answer A is incorrect, as lisinopril most commonly increases potassium levels secondary to its effects on the RAAS. The downstream reduction in aldosterone synthesis facilitated by angiotensin-converting enzyme inhibitors (ACEi) ultimately results in decreased sodium and water resorption at the expense of increased retention of potassium.[5,6]

Answer B is incorrect. Insulin can cause hypokalemia when used in the face of severe hyperglycemia due to dramatic glucose shifts that can occur moving from extracellular to intracellular spaces. However, AK's diabetes is fairly well controlled based on his hemoglobin A1c and serum blood glucose readings. Unless he was undergoing intensive insulin therapy for a condition such as diabetic ketoacidosis or hyperosmolar hyperglycemic state, it is unlikely that the sliding scale insulin utilized for treatment of his diabetes would result in hypokalemia.

Answer D is incorrect, as atorvastatin is not known to cause hypokalemia.

6. **Correct answer: C**
Rationale: In patients with HFrEF and NYHA class II–III symptoms tolerating an ACEi or ARB, current guidelines recommend replacement by an angiotensin receptor neprilysin inhibitor (ARNi) to further reduce morbidity and mortality. This recommendation came as a result of the statistically significant 20% relative risk reduction in the primary outcome of death from CV causes or first hospitalization for HF in patients receiving sacubitril/valsartan compared to enalapril in the PARADIGM-HF trial. The risk of angioedema is significantly increased with the use of ARNi in conjunction with ACEi. This reaction is facilitated by increased levels of bradykinin, a vasoactive peptide, imparted by both the neprilysin component, sacubitril, and the existing ACEi. Sacubitril/valsartan should be initiated following a washout period of at least 36 hours in patients taking ACEi to reduce the likelihood of angioedema. It should be noted that in patients receiving ARB therapy this risk is significantly reduced, and sacubitril/valsartan may be initiated when the next dose of ARB is scheduled.[10]

Answer A is incorrect. As noted above, concurrent use of ACEi and ARNi is contraindicated due to the increased risk of angioedema that can occur with use of both agents. Additionally, it should be noted that use of an ACEi with an ARB, not just in the combination of sacubitril/valsartan, should be discouraged due to increased likelihood of hyperkalemia and renal dysfunction. Answer B is incorrect, as beginning ARNi therapy less than 36 hours after discontinuing an ACEi constitutes as an insufficient washout period and can greatly increase the risk of angioedema. Answer D is incorrect, as it is not required to initiate sacubitril/valsartan in an inpatient setting because monitoring can be safely conducted by outpatient providers. It should be noted that sacubitril/valsartan can be initiated in an inpatient setting, provided patients have not taken an ACEi within 36 hours, are euvolemic, and have had electrolyte disturbances corrected.[10]

7. **Correct answer: B**
Rationale: The starting dose of sacubitril/valsartan is dependent upon the patient's current dose of ACEi or ARB. Patients established on a high dose ACEi (ex: >10 mg/day enalapril, >10 mg/day lisinopril, >5 mg/day ramipril) or ARB (ex: >160 mg/day valsartan, >50 mg/day losartan, >10 mg/day olmesartan) should be initiated on sacubitril 49 mg/valsartan 51 mg.[10,11]

Answer A is incorrect, as this dose is reserved for patients who are either naive to ACEi or ARB therapy or who are taking what are considered to be low doses (ex: <10 mg/day enalapril, <10 mg/day lisinopril, <5 mg/day ramipril or <160 mg/day valsartan, <50 mg/day losartan, <10 mg/day olmesartan) of those agents. It should be noted that this option could be considered if AK is not able to tolerate the dose of sacubitril 49/valsartan 51 mg.[10,11]

Answer C is incorrect as this dose is reserved for patients who have tolerated a minimum of the sacubitril 49/valsartan 51 mg. The risk of initiating the maximum dose of sacubitril valsartan without evidence of the patient tolerating lower doses of this agent could include possible hypotension, hyperkalemia, or acute kidney injury.[10,11]

Answer D is incorrect, as AK's renal function, potassium, and blood pressure are all within appropriate ranges where initiation of an ARNi would be appropriate.[10,11]

8. **Correct answer: B**
   Rationale: Completing the prior authorization process will allow his healthcare team to provide justification for the medical necessity of AK's new sacubitril/valsartan and ensure that he is able to obtain it from his Medicaid insurance at a reasonable price. It should be noted that eligibility for specific medications will vary depending on insurance carrier, as well as by state for Medicaid and Medicare patients.

   Answer A is incorrect as supplies of medication samples are often unpredictable and dependent on charitable or pharmaceutical representative donations. Answer C is incorrect, as drug manufacturer programs explicitly exclude patients with federal or state insurance policies, such as Medicare and Medicaid, from receiving benefits.

   It should be noted that a one-time 30-day free trial coupon could be provided to AK while his prior authorization paperwork and prescription are processed, but the coupon would not be considered a sustainable option if used by itself. Answer D is incorrect, as providing AK with a 30-day free trial coupon of sacubitril/valsartan will only be viable for one use, as patients are required to catalog their personal information with the manufacturer to prevent coupons from being issued repeatedly.

9. **Correct answer: A**
   Rationale: Four of the most common side effects associated with sacubitril/valsartan are hypotension (18%), hyperkalemia (12%), increased serum creatinine (2%–16%) or renal failure (5%), and cough (9%). Healthcare providers managing ARNi therapy should be diligent in monitoring vital signs, laboratory parameters, and patient-reported symptoms to identify if such adverse events are occuring.[10]

   As mentioned previously, neprilysin inhibition results in increased levels of bradykinin, which may result in manifestation of cough, as well as more serious but rare side effects related to angioedema. Both sacubitril and valsartan work to reduce blood pressure, which can possibly result in hypotension, making answers B and C, containing the possibility of hypertension, incorrect. Patients should be supplied with blood pressure cuffs to monitor the blood pressure at home, as well as be advised to monitor for symptoms such as dizziness or syncope. The ARB component of sacubitril/valsartan carries the possibility of elevating serum potassium levels, making answers C and D, containing the possibility of hypokalemia, incorrect. Furthermore, answers C and D are incorrect due to the fact that decreased serum creatinine is not an adverse effect of ARNi and would not be an indicator of impending renal impairment or acute kidney damage secondary to therapy.[10,11]

CASE 16

1. **Correct answer: A**
   Rationale: Vitamin K intake affects warfarin's effect, so a consistent amount of vitamin K in the diet is recommended to help RE maintain therapeutic INR levels.

While there could be a drug interaction between warfarin and a multivitamin that contains vitamin K, it would not cause fluctuating levels if RE takes her multivitamin daily. Since warfarin has a prolonged effect on INR, taking warfarin at different times of the day would not significantly affect RE's INR levels. Inconsistent exercise routines will not have a significant effect on INR levels.

2. **Correct answer: C**
   Rationale: RE has heart failure (1 point), hypertension (1 point), age 65–74 years (1 point), diabetes (1 point), stroke (2 points), and female gender (1 point). Anticoagulation with warfarin or a DOAC is recommended with a CHA_2DS_2-VASc score of 2 or more for women in the CHEST guidelines,[1] and a CHA_2DS_2-VASc score of 3 or more for women in the ACC/AHA guidelines.[1]

3. **Correct answer: A**
   Rationale: Direct oral anticoagulants (rivaroxaban, apixaban, dabigatran, and edoxaban) are recommended over warfarin for stroke prevention in patients with atrial fibrillation.[1,2] Rivaroxaban has the correct dosing for RE's renal function based on actual body weight. Aspirin is no longer recommended for stroke prevention in atrial fibrillation and enoxaparin is not used for stroke prevention as an outpatient. The dosing listed here for apixaban is for treatment of venous thromboembolism, though apixaban is commonly used for stroke prevention in atrial fibrillation due to its favorable safety and efficacy profile.

4. **Correct answer: B**
   Rationale. Rivaroxaban should be taken with the largest meal of the day, which is usually the evening meal. Patients should also be counseled to eat their meal and take their rivaroxaban at the same time every day. Dabigatran requires RE to keep her medication in its original bottle, and any remaining medication should be discarded 120 days after opening the container. Warfarin requires a consistent intake of vitamin K–containing foods, since vitamin K content will affect warfarin's effect.

5. **Correct answer: C**
   Rationale: To achieve rate control for atrial fibrillation, RE should be treated with a cardioselective beta-blocker. In addition, RE has heart failure with reduced ejection fraction, and only three beta-blockers (metoprolol succinate, carvedilol, and bisoprolol) have been shown to improve clinical outcomes. While atenolol and metoprolol tartrate are cardioselective, neither agent provides mortality benefit in patients with heart failure with reduced ejection fraction. Therefore, metoprolol succinate is the only choice that would be beneficial for both indications for RE.

6. **Correct answer: D**
   Rationale: Rate control is preferred over rhythm control for treatment of atrial fibrillation based on the AFFIRM trial.[3] Rate control is usually maintained with beta-blockers and non-dihydropyridine calcium channel

blockers. Amiodarone can be used for patients with heart failure and atrial fibrillation but would not improve these disease states. Amiodarone has rate control effects but would not be a better choice than other rate control agents. Amiodarone also has numerous adverse effects, including toxicities with the liver, thyroid, eyes, skin, and lungs, which limit its use. While there is a drug interaction with warfarin, this would not prevent the use of amiodarone.

7. **Correct answer: A**
Rationale: RE should be on a statin therapy due to her history of stroke and diabetes.[4] Since she is younger than 75 years, she should be initiated on a high-intensity statin based on the SPARCL trial.[4] Atorvastatin 20 mg is a moderate-intensity statin (which lowers LDL by 30%–50%), whereas rosuvastatin 40 mg is high intensity (lowers LDL levels >50%). This dose change would also help her reach the LDL goal of <70 mg/dL since she is at high risk for another atherosclerotic cardiovascular disease event. If RE were over 75 years, a risk-benefit discussion would be recommended to determine a high-intensity versus a moderate-intensity statin, since older adults can have more adverse effects with high-intensity statin therapy. Simvastatin 80 mg as a new initiation is no longer recommended due to a high risk of adverse effects, and ezetimibe is not recommended as monotherapy over statins.

8. **Correct answer: A**
Rationale: While direct oral anticoagulants require less frequent monitoring compared to warfarin, there are some laboratory parameters that should be monitored occasionally in order to ensure the efficacy and safety of therapy. Since rivaroxaban is cleared renally, serum creatinine should be monitored, and the dose should be adjusted once the creatinine clearance falls below 50 mL/min. Rivaroxaban does not require INR monitoring. Liver function tests (LFTs) can be ordered on an annual basis, but since RE has no hepatic problems at baseline, there is no need to order LFTs in 3 to 6 months. Rivaroxaban is not affected by pulmonary function, and it does not cause pulmonary dysfunction, so this monitoring is not required.

9. **Correct answer: A**
Rationale: The patient's prior to admission medications for management of her diabetes should be continued. Metformin is commonly held on hospital admission due to an increased risk of lactic acidosis with IV contrast. Insulin sliding scales allow for titration, as a patient's diet may change during a hospital admission. While the patient is on an insulin sliding scale in the hospital, it is appropriate to resume their home regimen for diabetes upon discharge, as the patient does not have any changes in renal function and does not appear to have poorly controlled diabetes which requires adjustment in medications. The atenolol should not be continued since this patient has heart failure with reduced ejection fraction

so the selection of beta blocker should provide mortality benefit (metoprolol succinate, carvedilol, or bisoprolol). Warfarin should not be continued for this patient due to poorly controlled INR and complaints about lab frequency. A direct oral anticoagulant would be a more appropriate choice for this patient.

10. **Correct answer: D**
Rationale: Comprehensive discharge planning anticipates and addresses barriers and patient-specific needs in advance of hospital discharge. Since we are switching her warfarin to Xarelto, sending her prescription to the pharmacy can help identify and address financial barriers before the patient leaves the hospital. Depending on the patient's Medicare coverage and her plan's formulary, we may need to initiate a prior authorization or consider switching therapies. Depending on hospital workflow, this may be completed by pharmacy, case management, social work, or the primary care physician. Some manufacturers offer copay assistance cards, but Medicare and other government plans are ineligible. This patient should also have an interpreter present when providing patient education. It would be valuable to identify if any additional caregivers or family members, such as her daughter, should be present for patient education, and coordinate accordingly.

CASE 17

1. **Correct answer: E**
Rationale: As asthma patients transition through the healthcare system, each transition is an opportunity to optimize medication therapy and reduce risk of adverse health outcomes. This will include reconciling medications, providing patient education, and identifying and addressing adherence barriers. Nonadherence to medications or expression that the patient may forget to take medications is a signal to discuss barriers to taking medications as prescribed. Even if the medication is unrelated to the disease state being assessed, it still provides insight into the lifestyle, habits, and difficulties in consistently adhering to medications. Answer B, regarding an asthma action plan, can be indicative of an adherence barrier because of a lack of understanding and knowledge regarding the consequences of poor asthma management. Patients who understand the potential consequences of poor control have a higher likelihood of adhering to medications and preventing adverse outcomes. Cost presents a very obvious barrier to adherence, as patients who cannot afford medications are limited in their ability to consistently take medications. Steroid inhalers may have a higher cost or copayment than albuterol and may be underutilized due to the higher cost and lack of perceived benefit compared to albuterol, which provides immediate relief of symptoms. While albuterol works quickly and effectively as a rescue inhaler, it does not address the underlying inflammation or provide long-term control.[1] A patient who states they do not always pick up their

inhaler due to cost requires assessment of a potential adherence barrier. This may require education on treatment goals and consequences of uncontrolled asthma, a discussion on the difference between rescue and maintenance medications, clearly defined expectations with each therapy including onset of action, and an assessment of cost issues. Patients may not feel the higher cost or copay associated with their maintenance therapy is justified if they do not see the value of that medication. Therefore, it is important to collect additional information from our patient to learn more about her adherence barrier, and address accordingly. Lastly, stating that albuterol makes the patient feel better indicates that the patient may not understand the differences between the two medications (controller and reliever) and therefore may not find value in a controller which does not provide an immediate feeling of relief. This being coupled with the cost as a barrier may explain why the patient prefers use of albuterol over use of an appropriate controller.

2. **Correct answer: B**
   Rationale: Ibuprofen is a nonsteroidal anti-inflammatory medication (NSAID). Aspirin and other NSAIDs can worsen asthma through inhibition of the enzyme cyclooxygenase-1.[1] When cyclooxygenase-1 is inhibited, there is a decrease in production of prostaglandins and an increase in leukotriene synthesis. Leukotrienes have a pathogenic role in asthmatic patients and therefore can lead to worsening of asthma symptoms and poor control. Propranolol is a nonspecific beta blocker. As a result, it can bind to beta2 receptors in the lungs, triggering bronchospasm. In addition to this, propranolol can block the effects of albuterol, a beta-agonist, thus preventing its bronchodilatory effects.[1] Both medications could be contributing to the severity of JR's flare. When reconciling medications, we can collect information from the patient on how frequently she takes ibuprofen and propranolol, since both are as-needed medications. If the patient requires them on a regular basis, and if they are contributing to worsening asthma, we can recommend an alternative or refer her to her primary care physician to discuss management of anxiety. The other answer choices are incorrect, as insulin therapy and antihistamines are not known to affect asthma patients directly. Antihistamines can in fact assist in asthma management if a patient is triggered by perennial allergies. It is important to evaluate her entire medication list when reconciling medications to ensure her home medications are not adversely affecting management of her asthma.

3. **Correct answer: B**
   Rationale: Answer A is incorrect. While this does represent an increase in JR's current therapy, it is still considered step 3 under the current GINA guidelines. Additionally, GINA recommends treatment with a long-acting beta2 agonist that has a fast onset of action (formoterol) in combination with an inhaled corticosteroid.[1] Answer C is incorrect as this would be a low dose ICS + LABA and would still fall under step 3 therapy. Answer

D is incorrect. Answer D represents an alternative maintenance therapy for JR's current therapy based on current GINA guidelines which no longer recommends SABAs as the preferred reliever. GINA guidelines recommend using an inhaled corticosteroid with formoterol as both controller and reliever of asthma. The decision has been made to increase JR's therapy to step 4, thus a medium dose ICS + LABA combination as controller and reliever is recommended.

4. **Correct answer: B**
   Rationale: Since this patient has diabetes, it is important to discuss the negative impact of frequent exacerbations requiring oral corticosteroids on her blood glucose management. Answer A is incorrect because overutilizing albuterol will lead to tachyphylaxis, or reduced response to albuterol, and will not address the underlying inflammation. Therefore, it is important to educate the patient on the necessity for maintenance therapy to control inflammation and prevent complications such as airway remodeling. Answer C is incorrect because it will take 2 to 4 weeks to see the benefit of inhaled corticosteroid therapy. It is important to set clear expectations and educate the patient on the value of rescue therapy and the benefit of maintenance therapy. Answer D is incorrect because all of the above are not accurate statements.

5. **Correct answer: C**
   Rationale: Comprehensive discharge planning should address whatever patient needs will support safe and effective care transitions. Our patient has already admitted to poor adherence due to issues with inhaler cost. Therefore, we can send her prescriptions in advance of discharge so that we can identify if cost will continue to be an issue. This may require changing her therapy, initiating a prior authorization if necessary, or providing supplemental copayment resources if available. We do not want the patient to continue to have poor adherence due to cost, as this will increase the chance of readmission and the associated costs to the patient and the healthcare system. Answer A is incorrect because JR should receive an influenza vaccination annually and a one-time dose of the pneumococcal polysaccharide vaccine based on her vaccination history and her asthma diagnosis. The pneumococcal conjugate vaccine is only indicated for patients ages 19 or older with a cerebrospinal fluid leak or cochlear implant, immunocompromising conditions, chronic renal failure, nephrotic syndrome, leukemia, lymphoma, Hodgkin disease, generalized malignancy, anatomical or functional asplenia, or individuals age 65 or older. Transitions of care provide an excellent opportunity to advocate for vaccinations, but we want to ensure we recommend appropriately indicated vaccines. Answer B is incorrect because healthcare institutions should provide information to the next-of-care provider to support continuity of care. This is not the responsibility of the patient, although we can certainly educate and engage them as well.

6. Correct answer: A

Rationale: Based on JR's vaccination history and also having a chronic lung condition (asthma), JR should receive an influenza vaccination annually and a one-time dose of the pneumococcal polysaccharide vaccine.[2] Answer B is incorrect as the pneumococcal conjugate vaccine is only indicated for patients ages 19 or older with a cerebrospinal fluid leak or cochlear implant, immunocompromising conditions, chronic renal failure, nephrotic syndrome, leukemia, lymphoma, Hodgkin disease, generalized malignancy, anatomical or functional asplenia, or individuals age 65 or older. Answer C is incorrect because the patient has an indication for pneumonia vaccination, and transitions of care are an excellent opportunity to administer vaccinations which will prevent risk of exacerbations, readmissions, and worsening patient outcomes. Answer D is incorrect because the vaccinations are not up to date at this time.

7. Correct answer: A

Rationale: At each transition of care, we must first collect information to guide our assessment and plan. Therefore, it is important to assess proper inhaler technique and medication adherence in patients to ensure her current therapy is optimized. Without adherence to prescribed therapy, patients with asthma are less likely to have symptom relief.[1] In addition to this, if patients are not using their inhaler therapy correctly, the medication(s) are less likely to have the desired effect and reduce symptom burden.[1] Answers B and C are not appropriate because we must first assess adherence, including her inhaler technique, to determine if she requires an increase in therapy or education on proper technique. Answer D is incorrect because follow-up is needed 2 to 6 weeks after we adjust therapy to evaluate efficacy. It is important to incorporate follow-up to provide continuity of care for patients.

8. Correct answer: A

Rationale: Proper technique is important to ensure patients receive optimal benefits from their inhaler therapy. For MDIs, the proper steps for use are found in answer A. If the patient breathes in too rapidly and with too much velocity, this can result in the majority of the medication being deposited in the back of the mouth and pharynx (answer B is incorrect). If patients do not breath out prior to using the inhaler, they will not be able to take a breath in after activating the inhaler. This would prevent the medication reaching its desired target, the lungs (answer C is incorrect). Patients should hold their breath for 10 seconds after use of their MDI. There is no advantage to holding their breath longer and this could possibly result in undesired bronchospasm (answer D is incorrect).

9. Correct answer: B

Rationale: Although JR's symptoms are now well controlled, it has only been 6 weeks since her medication was optimized. In the acute phase after an exacerbation, it is important to ensure that patients are not readmitted to the hospital or return to the emergency department for acute relief of symptoms. GINA guidelines recommend that patients be controlled for at least 3 months before considering stepping down therapy. Answer A is incorrect because the patient is well controlled at the moment and higher doses of medication are not warranted at this time. Answers C and D are incorrect as we need to maintain control for at least 3 months. Furthermore, when stepping down therapy, never step down more than one step at a time to ensure the patient does not suffer from a subsequent exacerbation.

10. Correct answer: B

Rationale: This patient's asthma is poorly controlled with her current therapy. This is evident by the need to refill her maintenance/rescue therapy prior to the date it is due. In order to reduce symptom burden and improve the patient's quality of life, a step up in her current therapy should be considered. Answer A is incorrect as it will not help to improve control of the patient's asthma symptoms. Answer C is incorrect. It represents an alternative treatment modality for patients who do not have access to ICS/LABA therapy or cannot tolerate it, but it does not address the need for more control of the patient's symptoms.[1] Answer D is incorrect, as long-term OCS therapy is not recommended for treatment of asthma due to OCS long-term side effects.

CASE 18

1. Correct answer: D

Rationale: Empiric antibiotic therapy should be initiated in adults with clinically suspected and radiographically confirmed CAP. Although procalcitonin is not a required test, the high procalcitonin indicates a high likelihood of bacterial infection.[1] Patients may also demonstrate leukopenia, and chest imaging helps confirm pneumonia.

2. Correct answer: C

Rationale: Cardinal symptoms of COPD include dyspnea, sputum volume, and sputum purulence. Typically, you need all three to start empiric therapy of antibiotics; however, if increased sputum purulence is one of the symptoms, you only need one other symptom. Mechanical ventilation (invasive and noninvasive) should receive empiric therapy.[1]

3. Correct answer: D

Rationale: *Streptococcus pneumoniae*, *Haemophilus influenzae*, and atypical bacteria such as *Mycoplasma pneumoniae* are all the most commonly identified pathogens with pneumonia secondary to a COPD exacerbation. Some patients who have frequent exacerbations, severe airflow issues, or mechanical ventilation may suffer from other pathogens such as gram-negative bacteria (e.g., Pseudomonas).[1]

4. Correct answer: A

Rationale: Regardless of exacerbation severity, the guidelines recommend all patients be on short-acting bronchodilators. Inhaled corticosteroids, long-acting inhaled beta2-agonists, and long-acting anticholinergics are utilized for long-term management but can be used during an exacerbation in combinations of a short-acting bronchodilator.[1]

5. **Correct answer: B**
   Rationale: When choosing treatment for patients, the main goals are to reduce symptoms and reduce the risk of exacerbation. When patients are on palliative care, it is imperative the patient goals change to enhancing the quality of life, helping patients with end-of-life care, and optimizing functions. COPD is chronic and worsens over time; therefore complete remission of disease is not possible.

6. **Correct answer: D**
   Rationale: Treatment for CAP should include a combination of beta-lactam plus macrolide or monotherapy with a respiratory fluoroquinolone for non-severe inpatient pneumonia. Patients who are allergic can use a beta-lactam with doxycycline.[1] Since the previous admissions were not within 90 days, MRSA coverage is not necessary.

7. **Correct answer: B**
   Rationale: Prednisone therapy has been shown to improve oxygenation, reduce treatment failure, and improve the length of hospitalization. The recommended dose is 40 mg daily for 5 days.[1]

8. **Correct answer: D**
   Rationale: Since the patient is already on a LABA + LAMA and has had multiple hospitalizations, it would be appropriate to start triple therapy with a LABA + LAMA + ICS. Answers A–C are not appropriate in this patient since he is already taking a LABA + LAMA combination therapy. Since the patient's eosinophils are >300, ICS additional may be helpful.[1]

CASE 19

1. **Correct answer: D**
   Rationale: Choice A is incorrect because the patient did not present with classic signs and symptoms of heart failure exacerbation such as shortness of breath and severe fluid overload. B is incorrect because while an unsafe home environment can certainly contribute to her falls, her overall presentation is better explained by low blood pressure and sedative state from overmedication as opposed to tripping over things at home. Choice C is incorrect as none of her complaints can be adequately explained by her chronic disease states. Choice D is the correct answer as her low blood pressure and her sedation are likely due to using multiple blood pressure medications as well as medications with central nervous system (CNS) effect.

2. **Correct answer: C**
   Rationale: Choices A, B, and D are all issues that should be addressed with WL. A is incorrect since trazodone has no apparent indication based on the past medical history

listed. B is incorrect since gabapentin is overdosed based on the patient's renal function. Using the Cockroft-Gault equation, WL has a creatinine clearance around 26 mL/min. Based on the package insert, gabapentin dose in patients with creatinine clearance between 15–30 mL/min should not exceed 700 mg/day.[1] D is incorrect since alprazolam is an inappropriate medication for chronic management of generalized anxiety disorder. Based on the guidelines, a selective serotonin reuptake inhibitor or a serotonin-norepinephrine reuptake inhibitor should be first-line for anxiety. Benzodiazepines should be limited to short-term use.[2,3] C is the correct answer since WL is on all of the medications with proven mortality benefit for her HFrEF at appropriate doses.

3. **Correct answer: F**
   Rationale: All of the listed types of medications can increase the risk of fall, especially in elderly patients. Blood pressure medications and antidiabetic medications may increase fall risk if the patient experiences hypotension or hypoglycemia, both of which can lead to falling. Anticholinergic agents can cause a myriad of adverse events including CNS effects such as ataxia, cognitive impairment, dizziness, sedation, and lightheadedness, which can increase the risk of fall. In fact, many medications with anticholinergic effects are included on the Beers list due to the risk of cognitive decline.[4] CNS depressants are medications that can cause adverse events such as drowsiness and daytime sedation, which in turn can cause falls.

4. **Correct answer: C**
   Rationale: A and B are incorrect because while hypoglycemia can certainly cause a fall, metformin and empagliflozin do not commonly lead to hypoglycemia. If these agents are combined with extensive alcohol intake, strenuous exercise, or poor diet, then hypoglycemia may result. Agents such as insulins, sulfonylureas, and meglitinides commonly lead to hypoglycemia based on their mechanism of action. In addition, her lab work shows that her blood glucose level is normal, and her diabetes is well controlled based on her A1C; thus these medications should be continued. D is incorrect because WL's physical examination indicates that she is slightly fluid overloaded as evidenced by pitting edema in her lower extremities and rales in her lungs. Additionally, there are no physical examination or laboratory values that indicate she is dehydrated such as decreased UOP, pale skin, dry mucous membranes, or constipation. WL does have low blood pressure, which can be a sign of dehydration, but she has overmedication that the hypotension may be attributed to. With these findings, it would be inappropriate to discontinue her furosemide. Trazodone should be discontinued since this is the only medication on her profile that has no apparent indication (abrupt discontinuation may lead to withdrawal symptoms, and discontinuation should be tapered). Trazodone is approved by the FDA for the treatment of major depressive disorder, although it is used off-label for insomnia, neither of which WL

is diagnosed with. Moreover, trazodone adverse effects include somnolence and fatigue, dizziness, hypotension and syncope, and hyponatremia, especially in volume-depleted and elderly patients or with concurrent diuretic therapy, which could contribute to her symptoms of lethargy and recent falls.

5. **Correct answer: D**
   Rationale: While all of the listed medications can potentially lower blood pressure, clonidine should be the first agent to be discontinued. A and B are incorrect because sacubitril/valsartan and carvedilol have compelling indications for patients with HFrEF, with proven mortality benefit.[5] C is incorrect since WL's physical examination indicated mild fluid overload, likely as a result of her HFrEF; therefore discontinuing furosemide is not appropriate. Moreover, furosemide's effect on blood pressure is likely mild. Clonidine should be discontinued first, not only because it is the only blood pressure drug WL is on without a mortality benefit, but also because it can have adverse effects, including hypotension, bradycardia, CNS effects, somnolence, and sedation. These adverse effects combined with other agents' adverse effects (e.g., trazodone) are likely what led to WL's fall and hospitalization. Clonidine should be tapered off to avoid rebound hypertension. Once this agent has been removed, we can reevaluate WL to assess her blood pressure, heart rate, fluid status, and symptoms of fatigue. We may then decide if additional agents should be discontinued or doses reduced.

6. **Correct answer: E**
   Rationale: All of the listed medications are on the American Geriatrics Society (AGS) Beers Criteria® for Potentially Inappropriate Medication (PIM). The AGS Beers Criteria is a list of medications that are potentially inappropriate to use in older adults.[4] Clonidine is on the Beers list for concerns for orthostatic hypotension, bradycardia, and CNS adverse effects. Gabapentin should be used with caution in patients with creatinine clearance of <60 mL/min or with concomitant opioids for concerns of increased risk of CNS adverse effects in renal impairment and risk of sedation and respiratory depression in patients on opioids. Benzodiazepines are listed for concerns for increased sensitivity and impaired metabolism, especially for long-acting agents, that increases risk of cognitive impairment, unsteady gait, psychomotor impairment, accidents, and delirium. Opioids like hydrocodone/acetaminophen should be avoided in elderly patients with a fall history. Opioids should not be used for chronic pain management in the elderly population and should be reserved for severe acute pain only (e.g., recent fractures or joint replacement). Lastly, antihistamines such as diphenhydramine cause anticholinergic effects such as confusion, cognitive impairment, delirium, dry mouth, constipation, and urinary retention.

7. **Correct answer: D**
   Rationale: A is incorrect, as NSAIDs would not be appropriate for WL given her poor renal function and her

cardiac condition. B is incorrect. Based on the Beers criteria, opioids may be inappropriate in patient with a history of falls or fractures (except for recent acute severe pain due to fracture or joint replacement), in patients on concomitant gabapentinoids or benzodiazepine.[4] C is incorrect as TCAs are not recommended due to lack of efficacy unless the back pain has neuropathic involvement.[6,7] Moreover, TCAs are not recommended for elderly patients based on the Beers criteria for adverse events such as anticholinergic effects, sedation, and orthostatic hypotension.[4] D is the correct answer. Exercise may provide a small improvement in pain and function. While type of exercise is not dictated, water exercise (e.g., aqua-jogging) may relieve pressure, and provides a low-impact option for exercise.[8,9] Multidisciplinary rehabilitation, which includes physical therapy, has been shown to provide moderate improvements in pain and small improvements in function.[9]

8. **Correct answer: A**
   Rationale: B is incorrect because spironolactone is not recommended in patients with eGFR of <30 mL/minute/1.73m² according to the heart failure guidelines.[10] In addition, the AGS Beers Criteria also suggests avoiding use in elderly patients with CrCl <30 mL/min due to concerns for hyperkalemia.[4] C and D are incorrect because both metformin and empagliflozin are renally adjusted based on eGFR. While empagliflozin does not need to be dose reduced, it is recommended to discontinue empagliflozin in patients with eGFR consistently lower than 45 mL/minute/1.73m².[11] Similarly, metformin is contraindicated in patients with eGFR of less than 30 mL/minute/1.73m², and hence should be discontinued.[12]

CASE 20

1. **Correct answer: D**
   Rationale: Medical respite care programs are offered in a variety of settings including freestanding facilities, homeless shelters, nursing homes, and transitional housing.[1] Medical respite care is an acute and post-acute care for people experiencing homelessness who are too sick or frail to recover from a physical illness or injury on the streets/shelters but are not sick enough to be in a hospital.[1] Medical respite care prevents unnecessary, costly hospitalizations and reduces hospital readmissions.[1] A study by Buchanan et al. found that patients who received respite care averaged 5 fewer inpatient days and a 36% reduction in emergency room visits during the year following their respite stay as opposed to patients who were denied respite care.[2]

2. **Correct answer: D**
   Rationale: According to National Health Care for the Homeless Council, poor health can cause homelessness if the patient is unable to afford housing due to the cost of medical bills or the inability to sustain a job due to medical illness.[3] As a result, patients may be displaced and without a home. Additionally, the National Coalition for the

Homeless reports that approximately 16% of patients experiencing homelessness suffer from mental illness. Lastly, individuals who experience domestic violence (women > men) are often forced to choose between abusive relationships and homelessness.[4] The National Coalition for the Homeless reports that domestic violence as a primary cause of homelessness in 50% of cities that was surveyed by the US Conference of Mayors.[4]

3. **Correct answer: D**
   Rationale: Pneumonia should be treated for a minimum of 5 days if the patient is afebrile and clinically stable; therefore, option A is incorrect as SS was only hospitalized for 3 days. On the other hand, it is very common for patients who are actively abusing substances to forget to take their medications when they are using, and thus there is a potential for SS to not complete his antibiotic therapy. Additionally, when patients are discharged, regardless of whether they are homeless or not, they do not always go directly to the outpatient pharmacy after discharge to pick up their prescriptions. This is commonly seen in patients experiencing homelessness. For someone like SS, he will most likely go back out to the streets and not pick up his remaining antibiotic therapy, which will result in a lapse in therapy. A meds-to-beds program or something similar will help reduce the delay in patients receiving their discharge medications.

4. **Correct answer: D**
   Rationale: SS has a history of getting disconnected to care. If patients are not seen for follow-up care, providers may not refill prescriptions because the patient is not being monitored properly. This is the case for SS when he was intermittently engaged with the methadone clinic and when he was lost to behavioral care. Additionally, patients experiencing homelessness are often living in the streets, and they carry their medications on them. Depending on where they live, the weather may get too hot, cold, wet, etc. As a result, improper storage of medications may compromise the integrity of the medications. On the other hand, SS has Medicaid so we are not concerned about not having insurance; thus, option B is incorrect.

5. **Correct answer: A**
   Rationale: Patient reported abusing alcohol/benzodiazepine to help cope with anxiety. You want to treat the underlying issue. If the patient's anxiety is controlled, they are less likely to abuse those substances. Although starting a medication-assisted therapy (MAT) for alcohol/benzodiazepine abuse would be appropriate for this patient, naltrexone is not appropriate. SS is taking methadone for opioid use disorder, so naltrexone will induce withdrawal symptoms for this patient.

6. **Correct answer: A**
   Rationale: For this question, it is important to understand the patient's co-infections, extent of liver damage, HCV genotype, and HCV viral load. This patient does not have HIV, and based on the FIB-4 score does not show evidence of cirrhosis. According to the AASLD guidelines,

ledipasvir-sofosbuvir is recommended in patients with genotype 1a (without cirrhosis) for 12 weeks.[5] However, ledipasvir-sofosbuvir can also be used in the same genotype for 8 weeks if the patient is not coinfected with HIV and has a viral load <6,000,000. Elbasvir-grazoprevir and sofosbuvir-velpatasvir can be used in this genotype but are both recommended to be used for 12 weeks and are therefore incorrect.

7. **Correct answer: B**
   Rationale: There is a significant drug interaction with Harvoni and PPIs/H2RAs that could result in decreased antiviral concentration and treatment failure. This can easily be avoided if the two medications are separated by 4 hours. A patient may be switched to interferon and ribavirin; however, it is not optimal as the patient is already 2 weeks into therapy and the DAAs have a much better ADR profile than interferon + ribavirin.

8. **Correct answer: D**
   Rationale: Many prescribers will prescribe a short-term medication supply until the next clinic visit or lab appointment. Some clinics may also have the ability to store patients' own medications. It is important to explore options available to the patient and assess which method would be most appropriate for your patient.

9. **Correct answer: C**
   Rationale: According to the AASLD guidelines, for patients who are NS5A Inhibitor DAA-Experienced (excluding glecaprevir/pibrentasvir failures) with genotype 1 regardless of cirrhosis status, sofosbuvir-velpatasvir-voxilaprevir or glecaprevir/pibrentasvir may help a patient achieve sustained virologic response (SVR) even after previous treatment failures; therefore, A is incorrect.[5] The recommended duration of therapy sofosbuvir-velpatasvir-voxilaprevir is 12 weeks; therefore, B is incorrect. Glecaprevir/pibrentasvir is recommended for 16 weeks of therapy and can be used to treat this cohort of patients as an alternative regimen, but the evidence behind this is somewhat limited. Therefore, D is not best answer.

CASE 21

1. **Correct answer: D**
   Rationale: Upon admission to the hospital, a best possible medication history should be collected. This includes a thorough history of all prescribed and over-the-counter medications, and should document medication name, dose, route, and frequency. Additionally, healthcare providers should assess adherence issues, barriers to adherence, and how the medication is actually being taken versus how the medication was prescribed.[1] Whenever possible, a patient interview should be conducted, and verified with at least one additional source such as a family member or caregiver, a community pharmacy, or a primary care physician. In this case, it is not appropriate to interview our patient due to altered mental status on

admission. Calling a preferred pharmacy can provide us with the patient's medication fill history but may not reflect any changes made to his medications, fill history from other pharmacies, or adherence issues. Similarly, information retrieved from the electronic health record will not always be comprehensive and reflect updates in therapy. In this case, the physician would be the best resource for current information on what medications the patient is taking. Once the patient is able to be interviewed, we can verify this information with the patient as well.

2. **Correct answer: C**
   Rationale: The RASS is a method employed by ICU clinicians to determine whether or not a patient is adequately sedated—another way to think of this is that the RASS score can tell how agitated a patient may be. The RASS ranges from −4 to +4, with lower numbers indicating heavy sedation or a comatose state, while higher numbers indicate increasing levels of agitation.[2-4] The CPOT score is used to quantify whether or not the patient is currently in pain, though it is important to note that this algorithm cannot specify the severity of pain.[2-4] The CAM-ICU screening tool is used to determine whether or not a patient has developed ICU delirium and takes the patient's RASS score into account.[2-4] Finally, the CHA_2DS_2-VASc score is used to determine the cardioembolic risk in patients with atrial fibrillation and is not relevant to this patient's presentation.[5]

3. **Correct answer: B**
   Rationale: The correct answer to this question revolves around the principle of analgosedation, which mandates that relief from pain should occur before providing additional sedating medications.[2] There are several reasons that this principle makes sense. First, a patient's agitation may be caused by pain, so it is very likely that a decreased RASS will be observed following the administration of an analgesic. Second, many analgesics are sedating in nature. By administering analgesics first, it is possible to address the underlying cause of the agitation without the need for administering additional sedating medications. Finally, if sedatives were administered first, or their doses increased such as the option with increasing propofol, it could mask the pain that a patient is experiencing.[2,6] Since this patient's agitation has been lasting for 3 hours, the best choice is to increase the continuous infusion of hydromorphone as opposed to a single dose of morphine. In addition, morphine has a relatively longer onset of action when compared to hydromorphone, meaning the patient would need to wait longer before experiencing relief.[6] Benzodiazepines should be considered a last-line option for sedation, as the drug class may be linked to an increased risk of developing ICU delirium.[2,8]

4. **Correct answer: B**
   Rationale: This is a complex opioid conversion case requiring multiple steps. The first step is to calculate US's hydromorphone use in the past 24 hours. Based on a continuous infusion at 0.7 mg/h, US has received 16.8 mg in the past 24 hours. While there are many strategies to opioid conversions, one of the safest ways to perform these calculations is to convert the current opioid dosage into morphine milligram equivalents (MME), and then from MMEs to the desired product.[9] Table 21-1 can help with equianalgesic doses and conversion factors.[10] In this case, IV hydromorphone has a conversion factor of 4 when converted to morphine equivalents.

   The first step is to make some relatively easy calculations through dimensional analysis:

   0.7 mg/h hydromorphone × 24 h = 16.8 mg total daily dose of hydromorphone

   16.8 mg hydromorphone × 4 (conversion factor) = 67.2 MME

   The following ratio and proportion can be used to convert IV hydromorphone to PO morphine:

   PO equivalent dose morphine = desired dose of PO morphine

   IV equivalent dose of hydromorphone = 24-hour dose of IV hydromorphone

   30 mg PO morphine = X mg PO morphine

   7.5 mg IV hydromorphone = 67.2 mg IV hydromorphone

   X = 268.8 mg PO morphine

   From this point, the dose of oral morphine can be easily converted to oral oxycodone:

   PO equivalent dose oxycodone = desired dose of PO oxycodone

   PO equivalent dose of morphine = 24 dose of morphine equivalent

   20 mg PO oxycodone = X mg PO oxycodone

   30 mg PO morphine = 268.8 mg PO morphine

   X = 179.2 mg PO oxycodone

   The hospital policy mandates a 25% reduction to account for incomplete cross-tolerance, which is the premise that patients may become tolerant to structurally similar agents over time, but such tolerance is thought to be incomplete.[11] In other words, a patient who is tolerant of an opioid would be tolerant to a different opioid, but that tolerance is incomplete in that a direct conversion to a full dosage of the second opioid could result in over-sedation and respiratory depression. Therefore, it is recommended to reduce the dosage of the second opioid by 25% to 33%.[11] In this example, 179.2 mg × 0.25 = 44.8 mg reduction, meaning the daily dose of oxycodone

Table 21-1. Morphine Milligram Equivalent Calculations*[,8,9]

Opioid	Conversion Factor (to MMEs)	Duration of Action (hours)	Dose Equivalent to 30 mg Morphine Sulfate
Codeine	0.15	4–6	200 mg
Hydrocodone	1	3–6	30 mg
Hydromorphone	4	4–5	7.5 mg
Morphine	1	3–6	30 mg
Oxycodone	1.5	4–6	20 mg
Oxymorphone	3	3–6	10 mg

*These estimates cannot account for an individual patient's response to therapy, given in part to unique genetic mutations in opioid metabolism and unique pharmacokinetics. Caution is advised.

Table 21-2. Select Analgesics and Sedatives in the ICU[2,12,13]

Medication	Mechanism of Action	Sedative Properties	Analgesic Properties
Propofol	GABA mediator	Yes	Yes
Hydromorphone	Mu-opioid agonist	Yes	Yes
Ketamine	NMDA antagonism	Yes	Yes
Midazolam	GABA agonist	Yes	No (minimal)
Dexmedetomidine	Central alpha$_2$ agonist	Yes	No (minimal)

GABA, gamma-aminobutyric acid; NMDA, N-methyl-D-aspartate

is approximately 130 mg. In addition, per hospital policy, 10% of this should be reserved for breakthrough pain. For ease of administration, this can be rounded to 120 mg of oxycodone for the total daily dose, with approximately 10 to 20 mg being reserved for breakthrough pain. Answer B is the only option that gets reasonably close to this requirement, as is common when taking product strength into account. Answer B provides for 120 mg of scheduled oxycodone divided into 4 doses, and 20 mg of oxycodone as needed for breakthrough pain available every 6 hours.

5. **Correct answer: A**
    Rationale: Regardless of whether or not patients have a similar request as US, it is important for clinicians to be well versed in multimodal pain management strategies. A rationale for treatment decisions can always be found by understanding the mechanism of action and clinical effects of medications. Dexmedetomidine is a centrally acting alpha$_2$-agonist that provides only light sedation and negligible analgesia and is primarily used in patients who require sedation after being extubated or to prevent them from being intubated in the first place.[2,12,13] Midazolam is a benzodiazepine that is sedating but provides only marginal amounts of analgesia. Though it was appropriate to titrate the propofol in option B to account for the additive sedative effects, midazolam is not an ideal choice for this patient.[2,12,13] Pentobarbital is an extremely potent barbiturate that is almost exclusively used when inducing a coma, and is not appropriate for this setting.[2,12,13] Ketamine is a NMDA antagonist that provides both sedation and analgesia and is becoming a drug of choice in ICUs in the current climate of opioid-sparing pain management.[2,12,13] Furthermore, as ketamine does have sedative properties, it is important to titrate the propofol accordingly. Thus, answer A is the best option. Table 21-2 provides relevant information for these agents with regard to their mechanisms of action and associated properties.

6. **Correct answer: D**
    Rationale: While all of these regimens provide multimodal analgesia, it is important to consider the specific factors that pertain to the patient and the complementary mechanisms of action of each drug. Option C is immediately incorrect due to the use of an opioid, and diazepam is a poor choice for a muscle relaxer when compared to the other options. Lidocaine patches have efficacy for localized pain; however, this patient's pain is likely coming from multiple areas considering the motorcycle accident, making topical lidocaine likely ineffective.[14] In addition, US has an open incision from his knee surgery, which is incompatible with lidocaine patches, making option A incorrect.[14] Ibuprofen is a nonsteroidal anti-inflammatory drug (NSAID) that can increase the risk of bleeding, which could be detrimental in a postoperative patient.[15] Furthermore, tizanidine is structurally similar to clonidine, so the use of both agents would likely result in dangerous hypotension, making option B a poor choice.[16] Option D is the best choice for US at this time, as it provides pain management for nociceptive (acetaminophen), neuropathic (gabapentin), and muscular (cyclobenzaprine) types of pain, in addition to the sedative properties of clonidine. Since dexmedetomidine and clonidine are structurally related and work on the same receptor, it is possible to infer efficacy of this therapeutic exchange. Published protocols regarding this scenario are available for review.[17,18]

7. **Correct answer: C**
    Rationale: Patients who have been immobile while in an ICU and on mechanical ventilation frequently have constipation. This is likely related to medications such as opioids but may also be related to their nutrition support. As a structural analogue of amitriptyline, cyclobenzaprine has potent anticholinergic effects that limit its usefulness in patients who may already have other risk factors for

constipation.[19] Other skeletal muscle relaxants also have anticholinergic effects, so it is important to choose an alternative wisely. Methocarbamol is not a potent anticholinergic and would be a suitable alternative.[19] Answers A, B, and D are incorrect because acetaminophen, clonidine, and gabapentin frequently cause constipation.

8. **Correct answer: B**
   Rationale: In order to answer this question, a thorough understanding of the PD/PK of US' medications is necessary. Typically, when antihypertensive medications cause hypotension, patients will experience reflex tachycardia to compensate. Dihydropyridine calcium channel blockers are notorious for this effect, although it is less frequent with amlodipine, likely due to its long half-life of approximately 36 hours.[20] Additionally, one would not expect amlodipine to be the main cause of hypotension in this patient, especially at one-quarter of the home dosage. Due to its mechanism of action as a centrally acting alpha$_2$ agonist, clonidine can cause both hypotension and bradycardia.[21] Furthermore, with a half-life of 12 to 18 hours, on day 3 of clonidine therapy, concentrations of clonidine are near steady state. Therefore, the dosage of clonidine should be reduced to 0.05 mg three times daily. Neither acetaminophen nor atorvastatin are commonly associated with hypotension and bradycardia, thus answers A and D are incorrect. Answer C is incorrect at this time because amlodipine is a medication that the patient was taking prior to his accident, while clonidine was only ever intended as a short-term medication for US.

9. **Correct answer: B**
   Rationale: The period prior to transfer to a SNF is a great opportunity to consolidate medications to only those that are needed. The patient is calm, so clonidine may be discontinued. The patient has not been on clonidine long enough to experience rebound hypertension, and the dosage of amlodipine is being increased to treat his underlying hypertension. The patient is improving otherwise, and methocarbamol may be decreased, with a goal of changing it to PRN muscle spasms. Pain control is adequate, so it is time to begin decreasing gabapentin, with a goal of discontinuing it when able to do so. Acetaminophen will still be necessary for pain control, with a goal of changing it to PRN pain. Atorvastatin should be continued. Thus, answer B is the best answer. Answer A is incorrect because clonidine is continued with no changes to his current regimen, and this option might delay his transfer to a SNF. Patients with limited mobility are at a greater risk of falls when taking diuretics, as the need to void the bladder may inadvertently force them to attempt to ambulate without assistance and may result in a fall.[22] The patient was on HCTZ prior to his accident, but since he is requiring assistance to get out of bed, it is not appropriate to resume diuretic therapy at this time. Thus, answer C is incorrect. Answer D is incorrect because completely removing

methocarbamol at this point might cause the patient to experience inadequate pain control.

10. **Correct answer: C**
    Rationale: At first glance, it may not be immediately recognizable that US needs any vaccinations at this time due to a motorcycle injury; however, a closer look at practice guidelines can help dissipate any uncertainty. The hepatitis B vaccine series would not be the most appropriate for US at this time since he is no longer using recreational drugs and he does not appear to have other risk factors at this time.[23] The zoster vaccination is not recommended in patients under the age of 60, though in some cases it can be used in patients older than 50. Regardless, US is 41 and not a candidate at this time.[24] Similarly, US is not within the target vaccination window for the human papillomavirus. Although some studies have shown benefit in a "catch-up" vaccine in patients up to 45 years of age, clinical guidelines do not routinely recommend this practice, and defer to clinicians to make the most appropriate choice for their patients.[25] The best choice for US at this time, based on the information available, is for a Tdap booster.[26] In 2020, the Advisory Committee on Immunization Practices updated their guidance document to allow for either Tdap or TD vaccines for wound prophylaxis.[26] Though the real concern in the case of compound fractures, like with US, is tetanus, the updated guidelines now allow for a booster of diphtheria and acellular pertussis as well.[26,27] Though the vaccination is most commonly administered in the trauma bay or emergency department upon patient presentation, it is always worthwhile to ensure that patients who have suffered compounded long bone fractures received a dose of either Tdap or TD prior to discharge.

CASE 22

1. **Correct answer: D**
   Rationale: Answer D is the best option because the pharmacist would be able to determine exactly when the patient last took a dose of clozapine. The patient has stated that he has stopped taking his medications, and his thoughts are disorganized and illogical because he is in an acute episode of schizophrenia. In this case, the patient may not be able to accurately tell the healthcare team when he last took his medications (answer A). Calling the patient's parents (answer B) could be an ideal option if the patient lived with his parents, but he currently lives in a group home. Calling the pharmacy that dispenses the clozapine (answer C) could be useful to determine medication adherence but will not tell you when the patient last took a dose.

2. **Correct answer: A**
   Rationale: Because the treatment with clozapine has been interrupted for more than 2 days, clozapine should be restarted at the starting dose of 12.5 mg once or twice

daily (rules out answers B, C, and D).[1] Starting at this low dose will reduce the risk of orthostatic hypotension, bradycardia, and syncope.

3. **Correct answer: A**
   Rationale: If clozapine treatment is interrupted for more than 2 days, it should be restarted at the starting dose to reduce the risk of orthostatic hypotension, bradycardia, and syncope (rules out answers B, C, and D).[1]

4. **Correct answer: B**
   Rationale: LM needs to be restarted on a starting dose of clozapine because his last dose of clozapine was more than 2 days ago. Clozapine 150 mg twice daily is higher than the recommended starting dose of 12.5 mg once or twice daily. If restarted at his home dose, LM is at higher risk for orthostatic hypotension, bradycardia, and syncope.[1] While clozapine does have a risk of severe neutropenia, restarting the clozapine at this higher dose does not increase his risk of neutropenia because neutropenia is not dose-dependent (answer A).[2] Clozapine does have a warning for hepatotoxicity, but this side effect is not associated with restarting clozapine at this higher dose (answer C).[1] Hypoglycemia is not a known side effect of clozapine (answer D).[1]

5. **Correct answer: D**
   Rationale: The pharmacist and other members of the healthcare team should work to improve medication adherence as much as possible by identifying factors that may influence adherence and addressing if possible. Because the orally disintegrating tablets start to dissolve in the patient's mouth immediately, it makes it more difficult for a patient to hold the medication and spit it out. Orally disintegrating tablets can be useful for patients who are inconsistent with swallowing medications.[3] Continuing to increase the clozapine dose every day without ensuring that the patient is taking it will increase the risk of orthostatic hypotension, bradycardia, and syncope, making answer A incorrect.[1] The patient was previously stable on clozapine, so a medication switch is not recommended at this time (answer B). In addition, LM has tried paliperidone unsuccessfully in the past. Answer C, continuing the starting dose of clozapine, does not help the patient and may extend his acute episode.

6. **Correct answer: C**
   Rationale: Clozapine may cause severe neutropenia. To reduce the risk of severe neutropenia with clozapine, the REMS program has a number of requirements. One of these requirements is ANC testing weekly for the first 6 months of treatment, every other week for months 6 to 12 of treatment, then monthly after 12 months of treatment. If clozapine treatment is interrupted for 30 days or more, the patient should be monitored as if they are a new patient with weekly ANC monitoring.[2] Because the patient's clozapine treatment has been interrupted for less than 30 days, the patient can continue monitoring every 2 weeks as before (answer C). He does not need to receive more frequent monitoring of three times weekly, or weekly (answers A and B). Answer D is incorrect because the patient has not been on clozapine for 12 months, so he is not yet to this monitoring frequency.

7. **Correct answer: A**
   Rationale: The new community pharmacy may not be certified in the Clozapine REMS program. If they are not certified, they will need to certify to purchase and dispense clozapine.[2] If the pharmacy does not complete the certification process right away, there could be a delay for LM in receiving his clozapine, which could potentially result in the need for re-titration of the medication and a reemergence of his symptoms. Verifying that the community pharmacy that will fill his medications is certified in the Clozapine REMS program will prevent this possible delay in care. If they are not certified, this gives them time to certify or to find another pharmacy if they do not want to certify. Group homes do not need to be certified to administer clozapine to patients (answer B). LM is going to be discharged on a higher dose of clozapine than when he was admitted to the hospital, so answer C is incorrect because the dose from his previous prescription would be too low. Because LM will not manage his medications at his new group home, he should not be the one who receives a paper copy of the prescription to bring to the pharmacy (answer D).

8. **Correct answer: B**
   Rationale: The amount of clozapine that can be dispensed depends on the monitoring frequency requirements from the Clozapine REMS program. A pharmacist should only dispense enough clozapine to treat the patient until the next blood draw or as directed by the prescriber.[2] LM's monitoring frequency is currently every 2 weeks, so the pharmacy should dispense a 14-day supply of clozapine (rules out answers A and C). The amount of medication that the insurance allows is unrelated to the Clozapine REMS program requirements (rules out answer D).

9. **Correct answer: C**
   Rationale: Patients who are nonadherent to psychiatric medications are at an increased risk for a relapse of symptoms.[3] LM should be counseled to continue his medications even if he starts to feel better (answer C). The monitoring frequency is not related to the dose or dose increases of clozapine (answer A). The prescriber or their designee can report the ANC results to the Clozapine REMS program.[2] If the pharmacist at the community pharmacy has the most recent ANC and it needs to be submitted to receive a "Predispense Authorization" (PDA), they can also submit it to the Clozapine REMS program.[4] However, LM's group home manages his medication, so LM should not be responsible for bringing the lab results to the pharmacy (answer B). Answer D is incorrect because the risk for severe neutropenia is highest in the first 18 weeks of treatment with clozapine, and it is not dose dependent.[2]

10. **Correct answer: D**

    Rationale: If a prescriber is not enrolled in the Clozapine REMS program, the pharmacist may use their clinical judgment and dispense clozapine to the patient if they provide a "Dispense Rationale" in the REMS program.[2] The patient must already be enrolled in the Clozapine REMS program and must have an acceptable ANC value on file.[2] The pharmacist should not dispense the clozapine without providing this documentation because the patient may not have an acceptable ANC value (answer A). Calling the new psychiatrist to inform her that she needs to become certified in the Clozapine REMS program is likely beneficial, but she does not need to be certified to dispense the current prescription if the pharmacist completes out a Dispense Rationale (answer B). The inpatient psychiatrist no longer treats LM and is no longer responsible for his clozapine. He would not be able to send another prescription for clozapine (answer C).

Standardized Laboratory Values

The following table is an alphabetical listing of some common laboratory tests and their reference ranges for adults as measured in plasma or serum (unless otherwise indicated). Reference values differ among laboratories, so readers should refer to the published reference ranges used in each institution. For some tests, both the Système International Units and Conventional Units are reported.

Laboratory Test	Conventional Units	Conversion Factor	Système International Units
Acid phosphatase			
Male	2-12 U/L	16.7	33-200 nkat/L
Female	0.3-9.2 U/L	16.7	5-154 nkat/L
Activated partial thromboplastin time (aPTT)	25-40 seconds		
Adrenocorticotropic hormone (ACTH)	15-80 pg/mL or ng/L	0.2202	3.3-17.6 pmol/L
Alanine aminotransferase (ALT, SGPT)	7-53 U/L	0.01667	0.12-0.88 μkat/L
Albumin	3.5-5.0 g/dL	10	35-50 g/L
Albumin:creatinine ratio (urine)		0.113	
Normal	< 30 mg/g creatinine		< 3.4 mg/mmol creatinine
Microalbuminuria	30-300 mg/g creatinine		3.4-34 mg/mmol creatinine
Proteinuria	> 300 mg/g creatinine		> 34 mg/mmol creatinine
or	or		
Normal			
Male	< 18 mg/g creatinine	0.113	< 2.0 mg/mmol creatinine
Female	< 25 mg/g creatinine	0.113	< 2.8 mg/mmol creatinine
Microalbuminuria			
Male	18-180 mg/g creatinine	0.113	2.0-20 mg/mmol creatinine
Female	25-250 mg/g creatinine	0.113	2.8-28 mg/mmol creatinine
Proteinuria			
Male	> 180 mg/g creatinine	0.113	> 20 mg/mmol creatinine
Female	> 250 mg/mmol creatinine	0.113	> 28 mg/mmol creatinine
Alcohol			
See under Ethanol			
Aldosterone			
Supine	< 16 ng/dL	27.7	< 444 pmol/L
Upright	< 31 ng/dL	27.7	< 860 pmol/L
Alkaline phosphatase			
10-15 years	130-550 IU/L	0.01667	2.17-9.17 μkat/L
16-20 years	70-260 IU/L	0.01667	1.17-4.33 μkat/L
> 20 years	38-126 IU/L	0.01667	0.63-2.10 μkat/L
α-Fetoprotein (AFP)	< 15 ng/mL	1	< 15 mcg/L
α-1-Antitrypsin	80-200 mg/dL	0.01	0.8-2.0 g/L
Amikacin, therapeutic			
Peak	15-30 mg/L	1.71	25.6-51.3 μmol/L
Trough	≤ 8 mg/L	1.71	≤ 13.7 μmol/L
Amitriptyline	80-200 ng/mL or mcg/L	3.605	288-721 nmol/L
Ammonia (plasma)	15-56 mcg/dL	0.5872	9-33 μmol/L
Amylase	25-115 U/L	0.01667	0.42-1.92 μkat/L
Androstenedione	50-250 ng/dL	0.0349	1.7-8.7 nmol/L
Angiotensin-converting enzyme	15-70 units/L	16.67	250-1167 nkat/L
Anion gap	7-16 mEq/L	1	7-16 mmol/L
Anti–double-stranded DNA (anti-ds DNA)	Negative		
Anti-HAV	Negative		
Anti-HBc	Negative		
Anti-HBs	Negative		
Anti-HCV	Negative		
Anti-Sm antibody	Negative		
Antinuclear antibody (ANA)	Negative		
Apolipoprotein A-1			
Male	95-175 mg/dL	0.01	0.95-1.75 g/L
Female	100-200 mg/dL	0.01	1.0-2.0 g/L
Apolipoprotein B			
Male	50-110 mg/dL	0.01	0.5-1.10 g/L
Female	50-105 mg/dL	0.01	0.5-1.05 g/L
Aspartate aminotransferase (AST, SGOT)	11-47 IU/L	0.01667	0.18-0.78 μkat/L
β$_2$-Microglobulin	< 0.2 mg/dL	10	< 2 mg/L
Bicarbonate	22-26 mEq/L	1	22-26 mmol/L
Bilirubin			
Total	0.3-1.1 mg/dL	17.1	5.1-18.8 μmol/L
Direct	0-0.3 mg/dL	17.1	0-5.1 μmol/L
Indirect	0.1-1.0 mg/dL	17.1	1.7-17.1 μmol/L
Bleeding time	3-7 minutes	60	180-420 seconds
Blood gases (arterial)			
pH	7.35-7.45	1	7.35-7.45
PO$_2$	80-105 mm Hg	0.133	10.6-14.0 kPa
PCO$_2$	35-45 mm Hg	0.133	4.7-6.0 kPa
HCO$_3$	22-26 mEq/L	1	22-26 mmol/L
O$_2$ saturation	≥ 95%	0.01	≥ 0.95

(Continued)

Laboratory Test	Conventional Units	Conversion Factor	Système International Units
Blood urea nitrogen (BUN)	8-25 mg/dL	0.357	2.9-8.9 mmol/L
B-type natriuretic peptide (BNP)	0-99 pg/mL	1	0-99 ng/L
B-type natriuretic peptide, N-terminal fragment (NT-proBNP)	0-299 pg/mL	0.289	0-29 pmol/L
		1	0-299 ng/L
BUN-to-creatinine ratio	10:1-20:1	0.118	0-35 pmol/L
C-peptide	0.51-2.70 ng/mL		40:1-100:1
		331	170-894 pmol/L
C-reactive protein	< 0.8 mg/dL	0.331	0.17-0.89 nmol/L
CA-125	< 35 units/mL	10	< 8 mg/L
CA 15-3	< 30 units/mL	1	< 35 kU/L
CA 19-9	< 37 units/mL	1	< 30 kU/L
CA 27.29	< 38 units/mL	1	< 37 kU/L
Calcium		1	< 38 kU/L
Total	8.6-10.3 mg/dL	0.25	2.15-2.58 mmol/L
	4.3-5.16 mEq/L	0.50	2.15-2.58 mmol/L
Ionized	4.5-5.1 mg/dL	0.25	1.13-1.28 mmol/L
	2.26-2.56 mEq/L	0.50	1.13-1.28 mmol/L
Carbamazepine, therapeutic	4-12 mg/L	4.23	17-51 µmol/L
Carboxyhemoglobin (nonsmoker)	< 2%	0.01	< 0.02
Carcinoembryonic antigen (CEA)			
Nonsmokers	< 2.5 ng/mL	1	< 2.5 mcg/L
Smokers	< 5 ng/mL	1	< 5 mcg/L
CD4 lymphocyte count	31%-61% of total lymphocytes	0.01	0.31-0.61 of total lymphocytes
CD8 lymphocyte count	18%-39% of total lymphocytes	0.01	0.18-0.39 of total lymphocytes
Cerebrospinal fluid (CSF)			
Pressure	75-175 mm H_2O	0.0098	0.74-1.72 kPa
Glucose	40-70 mg/dL	0.0555	2.2-3.9 mmol/L
Protein	15-45 mg/dL	0.01	0.15-0.45 g/L
White blood cell (WBC) count	< 10/mm³	10^6	< 10 × 10^6/L
Ceruloplasmin	18-45 mg/dL	10	180-450 mg/L
Chloride	97-110 mEq/L	1	97-110 mmol/L
Cholesterol			
Desirable	< 200 mg/dL	0.0259	< 5.18 mmol/L
Borderline high	200-239 mg/dL	0.0259	5.18-6.19 mmol/L
High	≥ 240 mg/dL	0.0259	≥ 6.2 mmol/L
Chorionic gonadotropin (β-hCG)	< 5 mIU/mL	1	< 5 IU/L
Clozapine, minimum trough	300-350 ng/mL or mcg/L	3.06	918-1071 nmol/L
		0.00306	0.92-1.07 µmol/L
CO_2 content	22-30 mEq/L	1	22-30 mmol/L
Complement component 3 (C3)	70-160 mg/dL	0.01	0.70-1.60 g/L
Complement component 4 (C4)	20-40 mg/dL	0.01	0.20-0.40 g/L
Copper	70-150 mcg/dL	0.157	11-24 µmol/L
Cortisol (fasting, morning)	5-25 mcg/dL	27.6	138-690 nmol/L
Creatine kinase			
Male	30-200 IU/L	0.01667	0.50-3.33 µkat/L
Female	20-170 IU/L	0.01667	0.33-2.83 µkat/L
MB fraction	0-7 IU/L	0.01667	0.0-0.12 µkat/L
Creatinine clearance (CrCl)	85-135 mL/min/1.73 m²	0.00963	0.82-1.30 mL/s/m²
		0.01667	1.41-2.25 mL/s/1.73 m²
Creatinine			
Male 4-20 years	0.2-1.0 mg/dL	88.4	18-88 µmol/L
Female 4-20 years	0.2-1.0 mg/dL	88.4	18-88 µmol/L
Male (adults)	0.7-1.3 mg/dL	88.4	62-115 µmol/L
Female (adults)	0.6-1.1 mg/dL	88.4	53-97 µmol/L
Cyclosporine			
Renal, cardiac, liver, or pancreatic transplant	100-400 ng/mL or mcg/L	0.832	83-333 nmol/L
Cryptococcal antigen	Negative		
D-dimers	< 250 ng/mL	1	< 250 mcg/L
Desipramine	75-300 ng/mL or mcg/L	3.75	281-1125 nmol/L
Dexamethasone suppression test (DST) (overnight), 8:00 am cortisol	< 5 mcg/dL	27.6	< 138 nmol/L
DHEAS (dehydroepiandrosterone sulfate)			
Male	170-670 mcg/dL	0.0272	4.6-18.2 µmol/L
Female			
Premenopausal	50-540 mcg/dL	0.0272	1.4-14.7 µmol/L
Postmenopausal	30-260 mcg/dL	0.0272	0.8-7.1 µmol/L
Digoxin, therapeutic (heart failure)	0.5-0.8 ng/mL or mcg/L	1.28	0.6-1.0 nmol/L
Therapeutic (atrial fibrillation)	0.8-2.0 ng/mL or mcg/L	1.28	1.0-2.6 nmol/L
Erythrocyte count (blood)			
See under red blood cell (RBC) count			
Erythrocyte sedimentation rate (ESR)			
Westergren			
Male	0-20 mm/h		
Female	0-30 mm/h		
Wintrobe			
Male	0-9 mm/h		
Female	0-15 mm/h		
Erythropoietin	2-25 mIU/mL	1	2-25 IU/L
Estradiol			
Male	10-36 pg/mL	3.67	37-132 pmol/L
Female	34-170 pg/mL	3.67	125-624 pmol/L
Ethanol, legal intoxication (depends on location)	≥ 50-100 mg/dL	0.217	≥10.9-21.7 mmol/L
	≥ 0.05-0.1%	217	≥10.9-21.7 mmol/L

(Continued on back inside cover)

Laboratory Test	Conventional Units	Conversion Factor	Système International Units
Ethosuximide, therapeutic	40-100 mg/L or mcg/mL	7.08	283-708 μmol/L
Factor VIII or factor IX		0.01	< 0.01 IU/mL
Severe hemophilia	< 1 IU/dL	0.01	0.01-0.05 IU/mL
Moderate hemophilia	1-5 IU/dL	0.01	> 0.05 IU/mL
Mild hemophilia	> 5 IU/dL	0.01	0.60-1.40 IU/mL
Usual adult levels	60 to 140 IU/dL	0.01	
Ferritin			
Male	20-250 ng/mL	1	20-250 mcg/L
		2.25	45-562 pmol/L
Female	10-150 ng/mL	1	10-150 mcg/L
		2.25	22-337 pmol/L
Fibrin degradation products (FDP)	2-10 mg/L		2.0-4.0 g/L
Fibrinogen	200-400 mg/dL	0.01	7.0-28.1 nmol/L
Folate (plasma)	3.1-12.4 ng/mL	2.266	283-1,360 nmol/L
Folate (RBC)	125-600 ng/mL	2.266	
Follicle-stimulating hormone (FSH)			
Male	1-7 mIU/mL	1	1-7 IU/L
Female			
Follicular phase	1-9 mIU/mL	1	6-26 IU/L
Midcycle	6-26 mIU/mL	1	1-9 IU/L
Luteal phase	1-9 mIU/mL	1	30-118 IU/L
Postmenopausal	30-118 mIU/mL	1	
Free thyroxine index (FT$_4$I)	6.5-12.5		
Gamma glutamyltransferase (GGT)	0-30 U/L	0.01667	0-0.50 μkat/L
Gastrin (fasting)	0-130 pg/mL	1	0-130 ng/L
Gentamicin, therapeutic (traditional dosing)			
Peak	4-10 mg/L	2.09	8.4-21 μmol/L
Trough	≤ 2 mg/L	2.09	≤ 4.2 μmol/L
Globulin	2.3-3.5 g/dL	10	23-35 g/L
Glucose (fasting, plasma)	65-109 mg/dL	0.0555	3.6-6.0 mmol/L
Glucose, 2-hour postprandial blood (PPBG)	< 140 mg/dL	0.0555	< 7.8 mmol/L
Granulocyte count	1.8-6.6 × 10³/mm³	10⁶	1.8-6.6 × 10⁹/L
Growth hormone (fasting)			
Male	< 5 ng/mL	1	< 5 mcg/L
Female	< 10 ng/mL	1	< 10 mcg/L
Haptoglobin	60-270 mg/dL	0.01	0.6-2.7 g/L
Hepatitis B surface antigen, extracellular form (HBeAg)	Negative		
Hepatitis B surface antigen (HbsAg)	Negative		
Hepatitis B virus (HBV) DNA	Negative		
Hematocrit			
Male	40.7%-50.3%	0.01	0.407-0.503
Female	36.1%-44.3%	0.01	0.361-0.443
Hemoglobin (blood)			
Male	13.8-17.2 g/dL	10	138-172 g/L
		0.621	8.56-10.68 mmol/L
Female	12.1-15.1 g/dL	10	121-151 g/L
		0.621	7.51-9.36 mmol/L
Hemoglobin A1c	4.0%-6.0%	0.01	0.04-0.06
		a	20-42 mmol/mol hemoglobin
Heparin			
Via protamine titration method	0.2-0.4 units/mL		
Via antifactor Xa assay	0.3-0.7 units/mL		
High-density lipoprotein (HDL) cholesterol	> 35 mg/dL	0.0259	> 0.91 mmol/L
Homocysteine	3.3-10.4 μmol/L		
Ibuprofen			
Therapeutic	10-50 mcg/mL	4.85	49-243 μmol/L
Toxic	≥ 100 mcg/mL	4.85	≥ 485 μmol/L
Imipramine, therapeutic	100-300 ng/mL or mcg/L	3.57	357-1071 nmol/L
Immunoglobulin A (IgA)	85-385 mg/dL	0.01	0.85-3.85 g/L
Immunoglobulin G (IgG)	565-1765 mg/dL	0.01	5.65-17.65 g/L
Immunoglobulin M (IgM)	53-375 mg/dL	0.01	0.53-3.75 g/L
Insulin (fasting)	2-20 μU/mL or mU/L	7.175	14.3-143.5 pmol/L
International normalized ratio (INR), therapeutic	2.0-3.0 (2.5-3.5 for some indications)		
Iron			
Male	45-160 mcg/dL	0.179	8.1-28.6 μmol/L
Female	30-160 mcg/dL	0.179	5.4-28.6 μmol/L
Iron-binding capacity (total)	220-420 mcg/dL	0.179	39.4-75.2 μmol/L
Iron saturation	15%-50%	0.01	0.15-0.50
Itraconazole			
Trough, therapeutic	0.5-1 mcg/mL or mg/L	1.42	0.7-1.4 μmol/L
Lactate (plasma)	0.7-2.1 mEq/L	1	0.7-2.1 mmol/L
	6.3-18.9 mg/dL	0.111	0.7-2.1 mmol/L
Lactate dehydrogenase (LDH)	100-250 IU/L	0.01667	1.67-4.17 μkat/L
Lead	< 25 mcg/dL	0.0483	< 1.21 μmol/L
Leukocyte count	3.8-9.8 × 10³/mm³	10⁶	3.8-9.8 × 10⁹/L
Lidocaine, therapeutic	1.5-6.0 mcg/mL or mg/L	4.27	6.4-25.6 μmol/L
Lipase	< 100 IU/L	0.01667	1.67 μkat/L
Lithium, therapeutic	0.5-1.25 mEq/L	1	0.5-1.25 mmol/L
Low-density lipoprotein (LDL) cholesterol			
Target for very high-risk patients	< 70 mg/dL	0.0259	< 1.81 mmol/L
Desirable LDL level and target for high-risk patients (optimal)	< 100 mg/dL	0.0259	< 2.59 mmol/L

(Continued)

Laboratory Test	Conventional Units	Conversion Factor	Système International Units
Above desirable	100-129 mg/dL	0.0259	2.59-3.34 mmol/L
Borderline high risk	130-159 mg/dL	0.0259	3.36-4.11 mmol/L
High risk	160-189 mg/dL	0.0259	4.14-4.89 mmol/L
Very high risk	≥ 190 mg/dL	0.0259	≥ 4.91 mmol/L
Luteinizing hormone (LH)			
Male	1-8 mIU/mL	1	1-8 IU/L
Female			
Follicular phase	1-12 mIU/mL	1	1-12 IU/L
Midcycle	16-104 mIU/mL	1	16-104 IU/L
Luteal phase	1-12 mIU/mL	1	1-12 IU/L
Postmenopausal	16-66 mIU/mL	1	16-66 IU/L
Lymphocyte count	$1.2\text{-}3.3 \times 10^3/mm^3$	10^6	$1.2\text{-}3.3 \times 10^9/L$
Magnesium	1.3-2.2 mEq/L	0.5	0.65-1.10 mmol/L
	1.58-2.68 mg/dL	0.411	0.65-1.10 mmol/L
Mean corpuscular volume (MCV)	80.0-97.6 μm³	1	80.0-97.6 fL
Mononuclear cell count	$0.2\text{-}0.7 \times 10^3/mm^3$	10^6	$0.2\text{-}0.7 \times 10^9/L$
Nortriptyline, therapeutic	50-150 ng/mL or mcg/L	3.797	190-570 nmol/L
Osmolality (serum)	275-300 mOsm/kg	1	275-300 mmol/kg
Osmolality (urine)	250-900 mOsm/kg	1	250-900 mmol/kg
Parathyroid hormone (PTH), intact	10-60 pg/mL or ng/L	0.107	1.1-6.4 pmol/L
PTH, N-terminal	8-24 pg/mL or ng/L		
PTH, C-terminal	50-330 pg/mL or ng/L		
Phenobarbital, therapeutic	15-40 mcg/mL or mg/L	4.31	65-172 μmol/L
Phenytoin, therapeutic (total concentration)	10-20 mcg/mL or mg/L	3.96	40-79 μmol/L
Phosphate	2.5-4.5 mg/dL	0.323	0.81-1.45 mmol/L
Platelet count	$140\text{-}440 \times 10^3/mm^3$	10^6	$140\text{-}440 \times 10^9/L$
Potassium (plasma)	3.3-4.9 mEq/L	1	3.3-4.9 mmol/L
Prealbumin (adult)	19.5-35.8 mg/dL	10	195-358 mg/L
Primidone, therapeutic	5-12 mcg/mL or mg/L	4.58	23-55 μmol/L
Procainamide, therapeutic	4-10 mcg/mL or mg/L	4.25	17-42 μmol/L
Progesterone			
Male	13-97 ng/dL	0.0318	0.4-3.1 nmol/L
Female			
Follicular phase	15-70 ng/dL	0.0318	0.5-2.2 nmol/L
Luteal phase	200-2500 ng/dL	0.0318	6.4-79.5 nmol/L
Prolactin	< 20 ng/mL	1	< 20 mcg/L
		43.5	< 870 pmol/L
Prostate-specific antigen (PSA)	< 4 ng/mL	1	< 4 mcg/L
Protein, total	6.0-8.0 g/dL	10	60-80 g/L
Prothrombin time (PT)	10-12 seconds		
Quinidine, therapeutic	2-5 mcg/mL or mg/L	3.08	6.2-15.4 μmol/L
Radioactive iodine uptake (RAIU)	< 6% in 2 hours		
Red blood cell (RBC) count (blood)			
Male	$4\text{-}6.2 \times 10^6/mm^3$	10^6	$4\text{-}6.2 \times 10^{12}/L$
Female	$4\text{-}6.2 \times 10^6/mm^3$	10^6	$4\text{-}6.2 \times 10^{12}/L$
Pregnant			
Trimester 1	$4\text{-}5 \times 10^6/mm^3$	10^6	$4\text{-}5 \times 10^{12}/L$
Trimester 2	$3.2\text{-}4.5 \times 10^6/mm^3$	10^6	$3.2\text{-}4.5 \times 10^{12}/L$
Trimester 3	$3\text{-}4.9 \times 10^6/mm^3$	10^6	$3\text{-}4.9 \times 10^{12}/L$
Postpartum	$3.2\text{-}5 \times 10^6/mm^3$	10^6	$3.2\text{-}5 \times 10^{12}/L$
Red blood cell distribution width (RDW)	11.5%-14.5%	0.01	0.115-0.145
Reticulocyte count			
Male	0.5%-1.5% of total RBC count	0.01	0.005-0.015
Female	0.5%-2.5% of total RBC count	0.01	0.005-0.025
Retinol-binding protein (RBP)	2.7-7.6 mg/dL	10	27-76 mg/L
Rheumatoid factor (RF) titer	Negative		
Salicylate, therapeutic	150-300 mcg/mL or mg/L	0.00724	1.09-2.17 mmol/L
	15-30 mg/dL	0.0724	1.09-2.17 mmol/L
Sirolimus (renal transplant)	4-20 ng/mL	1	4-20 mcg/L
		1.094	4-22 nmol/L
Sodium	135-145 mEq/L	1	135-145 mmol/L
Tacrolimus			
Renal, cardiac, liver, or pancreatic transplant	5-20 ng/mL	1	5-20 mcg/L
		1.24	6.2-24.8 nmol/L
Testosterone (total)			
Men	300-950 ng/dL	0.0347	10.4-33.0 nmol/L
Women	20-80 ng/dL	0.0347	0.7-2.8 nmol/L
Testosterone (free)			
Men	9-30 ng/dL	0.0347	0.31-1.04 nmol/L
Women	0.3-1.9 ng/dL	0.0347	0.01-0.07 nmol/L
Theophylline			
Therapeutic	5-15 mcg/mL or mg/L	5.55	28-83 μmol/L
Toxic	20 mcg/mL or mg/L or more	5.55	111 μmol/L or more
Thiocyanate	Toxic level unclear; units are mcg/mL or mg/L	17.2	μmol/L
Thrombin time	20-24 seconds		
Thyroglobulin	< 42 ng/mL	1	< 42 mcg/L
Thyroglobulin antibodies	Negative		
Thyroxine-binding globulin (TBG)	1.2-2.5 mg/dL	10	12-25 mcg/L
Thyroid-stimulating hormone (TSH)	0.35-6.20 μIU/mL	1	0.35-6.20 mIU/L
TSH receptor antibodies (TSHRab)	0-1 units/mL		0-1 kU/L

(Continued on back inside cover)

Laboratory Test	Conventional Units	Conversion Factor	Système International Units
Thyroxine (T$_4$)			
Total	4.5-12.0 mcg/dL	12.87	58-154 nmol/L
Free	0.7-1.9 ng/dL	12.87	9.0-24.5 pmol/L
Thyroxine index, free (FT$_4$I)	6.5-12.5		
TIBC—see Iron binding capacity (total)			
Tobramycin, therapeutic			
Peak	4-10 mcg/mL or mg/L	2.14	8.6-21.4 µmol/L
Trough	≤ 2 mcg/mL or mg/L	2.14	≤ 4.3 µmol/L
Transferrin	200-430 mg/dL	0.01	2.0-4.3 g/L
Transferrin saturation	30%-50%	0.01	0.30-0.50
Triglycerides (fasting)	< 160 mg/dL	0.0113	< 1.81 mmol/L
Triiodothyronine (T$_3$)	45-132 ng/dL	0.0154	0.69-2.03 nmol/L
Triiodothyronine (T$_3$) resin uptake	25%-35%		
Uric acid	3-8 mg/dL	59.48	178-476 µmol/L
Urinalysis (urine)			
pH	4.8-8.0		
Specific gravity	1.005-1.030		
Protein	Negative		
Glucose	Negative		
Ketones	Negative		
RBC	1-2 per low-power field		
WBC	< 5 per low-power field		
Valproic acid, therapeutic	50-100 mcg/mL or mg/L	6.93	346-693 µmol/L
Vancomycin, therapeutic			
Peak	20-40 mcg/mL or mg/L	0.690	14-28 µmol/L
Trough	10-20 mcg/mL or mg/L	0.690	7-14 µmol/L
Trough for central nervous system infections	15-20 mcg/mL or mg/L	0.690	10-14 µmol/L
Vitamin A (retinol)	30-95 mcg/dL	0.0349	1.05-3.32 µmol/L
Vitamin B$_{12}$	180-1000 pg/mL	0.738	133-738 pmol/L
Vitamin D$_3$, 1,25-dihydroxy	20-76 pg/mL	2.4	48-182 pmol/L
Vitamin D$_3$, 25-hydroxy	10-50 ng/mL	2.496	25-125 nmol/L
Vitamin E (a-tocopherol)	0.5-2.0 mg/dL	23.22	12-46 µmol/L
WBC count	4-10 × 10^3/mm^3	10^6	4-10 × 10^9/L
WBC differential (peripheral blood)			
Polymorphonuclear neutrophils (PMNs)	50%-65%	0.01	0.50-0.65
Bands	0%-5%	0.01	0-0.05
Eosinophils	0%-3%	0.01	0-0.03
Basophils	1%-3%	0.01	0.01-0.03
Lymphocytes	25%-35%	0.01	0.25-0.35
Monocytes	2%-6%	0.01	0.02-0.06
WBC differential (bone marrow)			
PMNs	3%-11%	0.01	0.03-0.11
Bands	9%-15%	0.01	0.09-0.15
Metamyelocytes	9%-25%	0.01	0.09-0.25
Myelocytes	8%-16%	0.01	0.08-0.16
Promyelocytes	1%-8%	0.01	0.01-0.08
Myeloblasts	0%-5%	0.01	0-0.05
Eosinophils	1%-5%	0.01	0.01-0.05
Basophils	0%-1%	0.01	0-0.01
Lymphocytes	11%-23%	0.01	0.11-0.23
Monocytes	0%-1%	0.01	0-0.01
Zinc	60-150 mcg/dL	0.153	9.2-23.0 µmol/L

[a]Hemoglobin A1c (mmol/mol hemoglobin) = (Hemoglobin A1c (%) − 2.15) × 10.929.

Source: Reproduced, with permission, from Chisholm-Burns MA, Schwinghammer TL, Malone PM, Kolesar JM, Bookstaver PB, Lee KC, eds. *Pharmacotherapy Principles & Practice*. 5th ed. New York: McGraw Hill; 2019.

INDEX